HAND
REHABILITATION
A PRACTICAL GUIDE

HAND REHABILITATION
A PRACTICAL GUIDE

Edited by

Gaylord L. Clark, M.D.
Assistant Professor, Department of Orthopedic Surgery
Johns Hopkins University School of Medicine
Attending Hand Surgeon, Raymond M. Curtis Hand Center
The Union Memorial Hospital, Baltimore, Maryland

E.F. Shaw Wilgis, M.D.
Associate Professor, Departments of Orthopedic Surgery and Plastic Surgery
Johns Hopkins University School of Medicine
Chief, Division of Hand Surgery
Director, Raymond M. Curtis Hand Center
The Union Memorial Hospital, Baltimore, Maryland

Bonnie Aiello, B.S., P.T.
Supervisor, Inpatient Physical Therapy
The Union Memorial Hospital, Baltimore, Maryland

Dale Eckhaus, O.T.R., C.H.T.
Clinical Specialist, Raymond M. Curtis Hand Center
The Union Memorial Hospital, Baltimore, Maryland

Lauren Valdata Eddington, R.P.T., C.H.T.
Clinical Specialist, Raymond M. Curtis Hand Center
The Union Memorial Hospital, Baltimore, Maryland

Illustrations by Joyce P. Lavery, M.F.A., A.M.I.

Churchill Livingstone
New York, Edinburgh, London, Melbourne, Tokyo

Library of Congress Cataloging-in-Publication Data

Hand rehabilitation : a practical guide / edited by Gaylord L. Clark
    ... [et al.] ; illustrated by Joyce P. Lavery
        p. cm.
    Includes bibliographical references and index.
    ISBN 0-443-08821-7
    1. Hand—Surgery. 2. Hand—Surgery—Patients—Rehabilitation.
    3. Arm—Surgery. 4. Arm—Surgery—Patients—Rehabilitation.
    I. Clark, Gaylord L.
    [DNLM: 1. Hand—surgery. 2. Hand Injuries—rehabilitation.   WE
830 H23275]
    RD559.H3597 1993
    617.5'7506-dc20
    DNLM/DLC
    for Library of Congress   92-49300
                                                            CIP

© Churchill Livingstone Inc. 1993

Distributed in the United Kingdom by Churchill Livingstone, Robert Stevenson House, 1–3 Baxter's Place, Leith Walk, Edinburgh EH1 3AF, and by associated companies, branches, and representatives throughout the world.

The treatment methods described in this text are intended to be guidelines for the therapist treating hand and upper extremity patients. It should be emphasized that these treatments and suggested postoperative timetables may vary depending on each patient's particular diagnosis and/or medical status. The therapist should always consult the patient's physician as to any variations in the surgical procedure or goals, treatment goals, and/or healing status of the patient.

Accurate indications, adverse reactions, and dosage schedules for drugs are provided in this book, but it is possible that they may change. The reader is urged to review the package information data of the manufacturers of the medications mentioned.

The Publishers have made every effort to trace the copyright holders for borrowed material. If they have inadvertently overlooked any, they will be pleased to make the necessary arrangements at the first opportunity.

Acquisitions Editor: *Leslie Burgess*
Copy Editor: *Elizabeth Bowman-Schulman*
Production Designer: *Patricia McFadden*
Production Supervisor: *Jeanine Furino*
Cover Design: *Paul Moran*

Printed in the United States of America

First published in 1993   7 6 5 4 3

We dedicate this book
to the founders of
The Union Memorial Hospital's
Raymond M. Curtis Hand Center:
Raymond M. Curtis, M.D.
E.F. Shaw Wilgis, M.D.
Gaylord L. Clark, M.D.
Frederik C. Hansen, Jr., M.D.
Rodney W. Schlegel, P.T., E.C.S.,
and
Janice Maynard, O.T.R.,
and to all of the hand
and upper extremity patients
past, present, and future.

Contributors

Bonnie Aiello, B.S., P.T.
Supervisor, Inpatient Physical Therapy, The Union Memorial Hospital,
Baltimore, Maryland

Mallory S. Anthony, R.P.T., M.M.Sc., C.H.T.
Senior Hand Therapist, Raymond M. Curtis Hand Center, The Union Memorial
Hospital, Baltimore, Maryland

Arlynne Pack Brown, P.T., C.H.T.
Clinical Specialist, Raymond M. Curtis Hand Center, The Union Memorial Hospital,
Baltimore, Maryland

Gaylord L. Clark, M.D.
Assistant Professor, Department of Orthopedic Surgery, Johns Hopkins University
School of Medicine; Attending Hand Surgeon, Raymond M. Curtis Hand Center, The
Union Memorial Hospital, Baltimore, Maryland

Dale Eckhaus, O.T.R., C.H.T.
Clinical Specialist, Raymond M. Curtis Hand Center, The Union Memorial Hospital,
Baltimore, Maryland

Lauren Valdata Eddington, R.P.T., C.H.T.
Clinical Specialist, Raymond M. Curtis Hand Center, The Union Memorial Hospital,
Baltimore, Maryland

Anne Edmonds, P.T., C.H.T.
Senior Hand Therapist, Raymond M. Curtis Hand Center, The Union Memorial
Hospital, Baltimore, Maryland

Beth Farrell, O.T.R.
Senior Hand Therapist, Raymond M. Curtis Hand Center, The Union Memorial Hospital, Baltimore, Maryland

Rebecca J. Gorman, P.T., C.H.T.
Senior Hand Therapist, Raymond M. Curtis Hand Center, The Union Memorial Hospital, Baltimore, Maryland

Gregory Hritcko, M.S., O.T.R., C.H.T.
Senior Hand Therapist, Raymond M. Curtis Hand Center, The Union Memorial Hospital, Baltimore, Maryland

Ann Leman-Domenici, M.S.W., L.C.S.W.
Senior Social Worker, Department of Social Work, Raymond M. Curtis Hand Center, The Union Memorial Hospital, Baltimore, Maryland

Barbara Rabinowitz, O.T.R., C.H.T.
Senior Hand Therapist, Raymond M. Curtis Hand Center, The Union Memorial Hospital, Baltimore, Maryland

Lorie Theisen, O.T.R., C.H.T.
Clinical Specialist, Raymond M. Curtis Hand Center, The Union Memorial Hospital, Baltimore, Maryland

Linda Coll Ware, O.T.R.
Occupational Therapist, Raymond M. Curtis Hand Center, The Union Memorial Hospital, Baltimore, Maryland

E.F. Shaw Wilgis, M.D.
Associate Professor, Departments of Orthopedic Surgery and Plastic Surgery, Johns Hopkins University School of Medicine; Chief, Division of Hand Surgery, and Director, Raymond M. Curtis Hand Center, The Union Memorial Hospital, Baltimore, Maryland

Foreword

The impetus for my becoming a hand surgeon started with Raymond M. Curtis twenty years ago during my residency at Johns Hopkins Hospital. Dr. Curtis, one of the pioneers in hand surgery, emphasized meticulous preoperative planning, precise surgical technique, and the importance of hand rehabilitation. Before the advent of hand therapy as a specific discipline, he spent many hours performing therapy on his own patients, both preoperatively and postoperatively. Through his vision, The Union Memorial Hospital created the Hand Center, one of the first hand rehabilitation centers in the world, with a staff of outstanding surgeons dedicated to surgery of the hand.

After Dr. Curtis retired, the Hand Center continued to grow and develop under the direction of Drs. Shaw Wilgis and Gaylord Clark. Today, the Raymond M. Curtis Hand Center is recognized worldwide as a center of innovation and excellence in the rehabilitation of hand disorders. Among its accomplishments are the work evaluation protocols and the BTE work simulator that were developed there.

It is an honor for me to write the foreword for this text, *Hand Rehabilitation: A Practical Guide*, for it is Drs. Curtis, Wilgis, and Clark who were my mentors. Learning the indications for and how to perform hand surgery is, however, only one-half of the equation. Hand therapy preoperatively and postoperatively is the most critical factor in achieving the best possible results for our patients. It is through Bonnie Aiello, Dale Eckhaus, and Lauren Valdata Eddington that I learned these principles.

Based on over twenty years of experience, the authors have written a practical guide to hand rehabilitation of commonly seen disorders. The 43 individual chapters start with basic principles of wound management, sensory evaluation, desensitization, and sensory re-education. Each chapter is organized alike, with an introduction, treatment purposes, goals, and indications and techniques for nonoperative and postoperative therapy. Each chapter provides for each topic a list of possible complications to alert the therapist, followed by an evaluation timetable to measure the patient's progress. Each chapter concludes with a current bibliography and suggested readings. The staff at The Union Memorial Hospital has performed a great service to the field of hand surgery by providing therapists, surgeons, and hand fellows with practical and useful guidelines we can all use in pursuing our goal of achieving the best possible functional results for our patients with disorders of the hand and upper extremity.

Andrew J. Weiland, M.D.
Surgeon in Chief
The Hospital for Special Surgery
Professor
Divisions of Orthopaedics and Plastic Surgery
Department of Surgery
Cornell University Medical College
New York, New York

Preface

Hand Rehabilitation: A Practical Guide began as a small-scale project and grew into a department-wide endeavor involving the hand therapists and hand surgeons at the Raymond M. Curtis Hand Center. It originated from our own need to organize the vast amount of valuable information we have gathered from being part of such a unique setting. Our purpose was to create a valuable teaching tool for new graduates, hand fellows, hand therapists, and surgeons that would relate therapeutic approaches to various diagnoses.

The book is designed to provide guidelines and a stimulus for therapists to analyze diagnoses of hand and upper extremity patients. We do not want this book to be viewed as a "protocol" to treat, or a "cookbook" for the non-professional to "follow directions." It is to be an adjunct to one's knowledge, a guideline for different treatment methods, and a resource for information. The information provided and the format it is presented in can be used in a number of treatment settings. The book is an educational tool to be used in combination with the knowledge and training of the professional.

We hope our goal of providing a method of quality care for hand and upper extremity patients is achieved.

The Editors and Authors

Acknowledgments

The editors and contributors thank Nancy Frisk Millner for her tireless patience and expert help in preparing our manuscript from our initial drafts to the completed project. Without her assistance, the preparation of this book would have been nearly impossible.

Peter Andrews is thanked for his photographic expertise and his flexibility in working with us.

Dr. Michael A. McClinton, Dr. J. Russell Moore, Dr. Anne B. Redfern, and Dr. Neal B. Zimmerman are thanked for their reviews and critiques of the manuscript drafts.

The therapists would like to thank Dr. Gaylord L. Clark for his contribution of surgical procedures to the chapters of this book.

Contents

Wounds

1

Mallory S. Anthony

Those of us involved with the treatment of hand injuries know how detrimental even a small wound can be to hand function. Almost all hand structures are made up of dense connective tissue, and essential to normal hand function is the ability of these strong connective tissue structures to glide in relation to one another. The formation of scar tissue after wounding can significantly impede gliding and thus decrease function. A thorough understanding of wound management throughout all phases of wound healing (i.e., inflammation, fibroplasia, epithelialization, contraction, and scar maturation) is important in developing a comprehensive treatment program.

During the initial phases of wound healing, we must concentrate on the preservation of function by preventing edema and subsequent fibrosis, as well as maintaining gliding surfaces. We must facilitate wound closure based on our knowledge of wound healing and effective dressing techniques.

During the final phases of wound healing, the scar maturation phase, our role is to apply controlled stress to the scar, thereby increasing gliding potential and allowing the most functional outcome.

The following guideline suggests evaluation and wound care techniques that should help the clinician expedite wound closure, minimize scar formation, and achieve optimum functional results.

DEFINITION

A disruption of the anatomic or functional continuity of tissue

I. Wound classification
   A. Tidy wound: clean laceration, minimal tissue damage, minimal contamination (Fig. 1-1A).

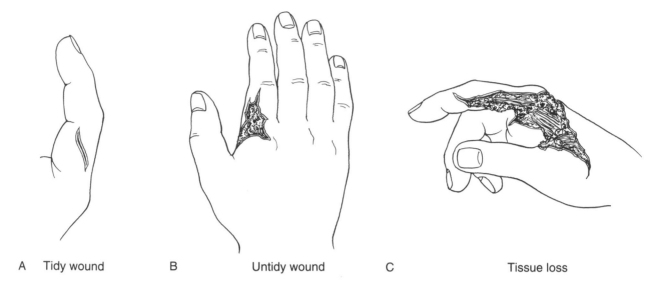

A   Tidy wound   B   Untidy wound   C   Tissue loss

Fig. 1-1(A). Tidy wound, **(B)** untidy wound, and **(C)** wound with tissue loss.

B. Untidy wound: significant amount of tissue damage (e.g., crush injury), uncertainty regarding viability of deeper structures, may have higher degree of contamination (Fig. 1-1B).

C. Wound with tissue loss: deeper vital structures may be involved (vessels, tendon, nerve, bone); may require soft tissue coverage (Fig. 1-1C).

   1. Split-thickness skin grafts (STSG) (epidermis and part of dermis) or full-thickness (FTSG) (epidermis and entire underlying dermis): replace skin in areas where adequate subcutaneous tissues remain to protect underlying parts and vascularize the graft.

   2. Flap coverage is necessary when the wound bed has exposed vital structures or when the bed has either a poor chance or no chance of providing vascularization for a graft.

D. Infected wound: presently or potentially infected.

SURGICAL PURPOSE

To achieve complete healing of soft tissue, to minimize scar formation, and allow for the maximum function of the underlying anatomic components (e.g., tendon, nerve, blood vessels, bone, etc.).

TREATMENT GOAL

I. Promote wound closure as quickly as possible with minimal scar formation.

II. Restore active range of motion (AROM) and passive range of motion

(PROM) in involved area, through scar management and range of
motion (ROM) exercises.
III. Maintain full ROM of all uninvolved joints of the upper extremity.
IV. Return to previous level of function.

INDICATIONS/PRECAUTIONS FOR THERAPY

I. Indications
  A. Primary closure: immediate wound closure, for example, tidy
     wound (sutures, grafts).
  B. Delayed primary closure: wound left open following injury be-
     cause the degree of bacterial contamination or the extent of vascu-
     lar impairment is in doubt (usually left open 4 to 5 days, then closed
     with minimal risk of infection), for example, untidy wounds.
  C. Secondary intention: wound closes through natural biologic pro-
     cesses of epithelialization, inflammation, fibroplasia, scar matura-
     tion, and contraction. Commonly employed for heavily contami-
     nated wounds and for extensive superficial wounds with tissue loss.
II. Precautions
  A. Infection
  B. Damage to deep vital structures
  C. Extreme pain
  D. Severe edema

THERAPY

I. Pretreatment evaluation
  A. Wound history
     1. Mechanism, force, duration of injury
     2. Time interval between injury and onset of treatment: acute
        versus chronic
  B. Patient history
     1. Age
     2. Occupation and avocational interests
     3. Alcohol, tobacco, or caffeine use
     4. Metabolic status: underlying disease affecting circulation (i.e.,
        diabetes, vascular disorders)
     5. Nutritional status
     6. Medications (i.e., steroids, anticoagulants)
  C. Subjective evaluation
     1. Pain (location, description, frequency, what relieves pain,
        etc.)
  D. Objective wound evaluation
     1. General inspection of upper extremity
        a. Edema

          b. Color
          c. Temperature
      2. Location of wound
          a. Anatomic landmarks
      3. Wound classification
          a. Primary/delayed primary
          b. Secondary
      4. Configuration
          a. Size
          b. Shape
          c. Depth (can use sterile cotton-tipped applicator)
      5. Inflammatory response
          a. Normal (5 to 7 days, up to 2 weeks)
          b. Prolonged or abnormal (2 to 4 weeks or longer)
             i. Infection (edema, redness, warmth, pain)
            ii. Cellulitis (redness and edema extending well beyond wound boundaries)
           iii. Lymphangitis (streaking redness)
           iv. Venous obstruction (cyanotic blue appearance of surrounding skin)
            v. Arterial insufficiency (pallor of surrounding skin)
      6. Maceration
      7. Exudate characteristics
          a. Color
          b. Odor
          c. Consistency (thin serous, purulent and viscous)
      8. Wound bed
          a. Color and extent of granulation tissue (red wound)
          b. Presence of epithelial budding (small pink islets forming within the wound)
          c. Presence of adherent fibrinous exudate and debris (yellow wound)
          d. Presence of dark, thick eschar (black wound)
      9. Other observations
          a. Degree of hydration
          b. Temperature
          c. Exposure of vital structures
II. Wound management
   A. Debridement and cleansing to assist in removal of exudate and necrotic tissue, decrease surface contamination, and control wound pathogens[1]
      1. Whirlpool
          a. Debrides superficial necrotic material.
          b. Recommended temperature is 94°F to 98°F (higher temperatures may increase edema).[2]
          c. Degree of agitation and duration depends on viability of tissues and patient comfort.

        d. Also creates sedation and analgesic effect (may aid in decreasing pain).

        e. Additives: at present no meaningful data exist to substantiate the therapeutic benefit of additives. Also, povidone–iodine and sodium hypochlorite, common additives, can be cytotoxic if not diluted properly.[1]

  2. Irrigation

        a. Debrides superficial necrotic material.

        b. Uses sterile water or antiseptic solution in water pik or syringe to flush out wound.

        c. Not a commonly used method.

  3. Debridement

        a. Selective (removes only necrotic material).

            i. Topical application of enzymes (Travase, Elase, Collagenase).

            ii. Manual debridement with surgical instruments. Care must be taken not to disturb delicate granulation tissue and migrating epithelium at wound margins.

            iii. Autolytic debridement (self-digestion of necrotic tissue by enzymes naturally present in wound fluids; facilitated by synthetic occlusive dressings.[1]

        b. Nonselective debridement (removes both nonviable and viable tissue from the wound; chosen for wounds containing excessive necrotic tissue).

            i. Wet to dry dressings. Be careful not to remove new epithelium and granulation tissue when removing these dressings.

            ii. Whirlpool or irrigation.

            iii. Hydrogen peroxide. Use with care—foaming effervescence may wash away healthy tissue. May be more cytotoxic than bactericidal.[1] Mainly used to help loosen dried exudate or debris.

B. Dressings

  1. Purpose

        a. Provide physiologic environment for wound

        b. Protect from further trauma and bacterial contamination

        c. Antisepsis

        d. Pressure to help decrease edema

        e. Immobilization

        f. Debridement if needed

  2. Components

        a. Contact layer: dry, adherent, or nonadherent

        b. Intermediate layer: absorptive, protective, and supportive

        c. Outer layer: holds dressing in place

  3. Types

        a. Adherent dressing used when amount of necrotic tissue is greater than viable tissue and debridement is necessary.

Necrotic tissue is debrided when the dressings *are re-moved*.

   i. Wet to dry dressing: saline-soaked sterile gauze placed directly on wound, then covered with dry gauze pads and outer wrap (Fig. 1-2).
   ii. Wet to wet dressing: same as wet to dry, except the dressing is periodically soaked with more saline to keep it moist (Fig. 1-3).
b. Non-adherent dressing used on tidy wounds (i.e., surgical incision, donor site) and open wounds composed primarily of viable granulation tissue, to minimize tissue disruption (Fig. 1-4).
   i. Vaseline gauze
   ii. Adaptic
   iii. Xeroform
c. Permeable dressing used for draining wounds: dry dressing with secondary absorbent layer to draw wound secretions away by capillary action (Fig. 1-5).
d. Occlusive dressing
   i. Provides moist environment and expedites rate of epithelialization, but may create an environment more conducive to maceration and increased bacterial proliferation. Use only on clean granulation tissue (Fig. 1-6).
   ii. Many types available including semipermeables, hydrogels, and biosynthetics.[3]
e. Wound packing: used with large deep wounds, when su-

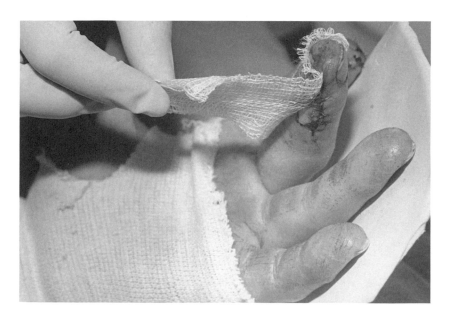

Fig. 1-2. Wet to dry dressing.

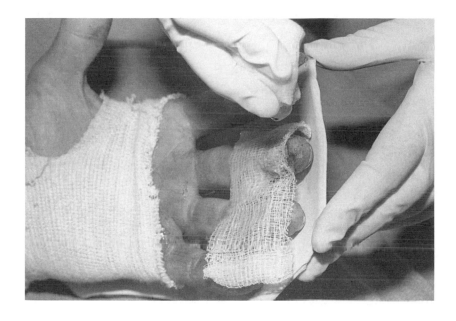

Fig. 1-3. Wet to wet dressing.

perficial portions of wound need to be kept open. Tight packing may cause ischemia.[3]

C. Topical agents
    1. Mercurochrome (5 percent solution): liquid antibacterial agent applied to small open areas to promote drying; usually left open.
    2. Silver nitrate ($AgNO_3$): applied with a stick and rolled across hypertrophic granulation tissue to cauterize and flatten this

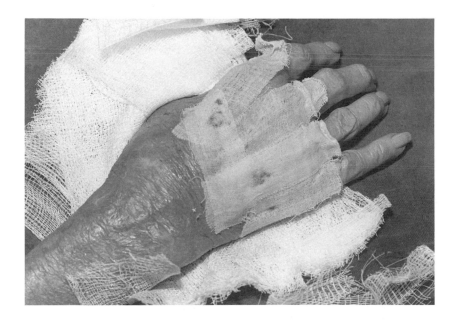

Fig. 1-4. Nonadherent dressing.

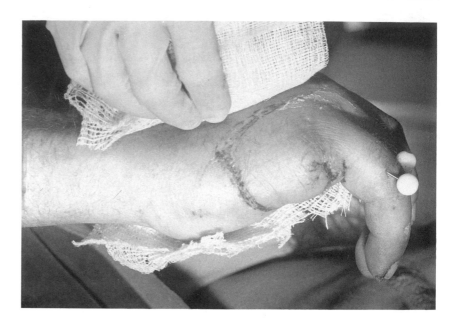

Fig. 1-5. Dry dressing.

raised tissue. (Please note this form of AgNO$_3$ should be distinguished from the 0.5 antimicrobial solution, frequently used for burn wound care). Table salt may also be used to flatten hypertrophic granulation tissue.

3. Silvadene: antimicrobial agent; bacteriostatic; keeps eschar soft and wound from drying.[1,3]
4. Povidone–iodine: good antimicrobial action, but cytotoxic effects.[1,3]
5. Bacitracin and Neosporin: antimicrobial agents; provide moist environment for dry wounds.

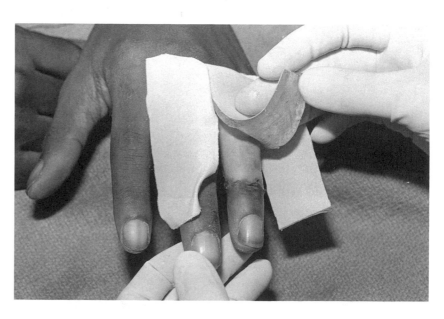

Fig. 1-6. Occlusive dressings.

D. Choice of dressing changes as wound status changes.

E. If wound is clean and healing well, topical antimicrobial agents are not needed. However, if wound is heavily contaminated and needs to be disinfected, use topical antibiotics (e.g., Silvadene [silver sulfadiazine], Neosporin, bacitracin) as opposed to antiseptics (e.g. povodine-iodine, hydrogen peroxide, boric acid, alcohols, chlorohexidene, merthiolate), which may be cytotoxic.[4]

F. Patients may do daily dressing changes at home, depending on their reliability and severity of their wound.

III. Early therapeutic intervention
    A. Edema control
        1. Effects of edema on wound healing
            a. Decreases arterial, venous, and lymphatic flow.
            b. Increases risk of infection.
            c. Decreases motion, which could lead to permanent tissue shortening and fibrosis.
        2. Therapeutic management of edema
            a. Elevation
            b. ROM exercise (combined with elevation)
            c. Intermittent compression
                i. Fluid flushing massage
                ii. Vasopneumatic devices (e.g., Jobst)
                iii. String wrapping
            d. Continuous compression
                i. Coban wraps
                ii. Ace wraps
                iii. Compressive garments (Jobst, tubigrip, Isotoner gloves)
                iv. Air splints
            e. Thermal agents
                i. Moist heat in elevated position (after inflammatory phase)
                ii. Cryotherapy for acute edema
            f. Microdyne
    B. ROM
        1. Maintain ROM in uninvolved joints
        2. Prevent remodeling of scar in shortened position
    C. Splinting
        1. Early protective splinting
            a. Avoid undue stress to wound and healing structures.
            b. Decrease development of shortened remodeled scar.
    D. Pain management

IV. Late therapeutic intervention (scar management)
    A. Pharmacologic (colchicine, betaaminoproprionitrile (BAPN)—clinical application limited at present)
    B. Mechanical
        1. Surgical excision
        2. Skin grafting
        3. Therapeutic application of stress (to realign collagen fibers

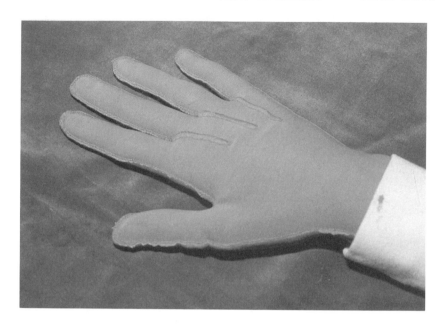

Fig. 1-7. Compressive garment.

in a more orderly and parallel configuration; application of pressure to theoretically decrease vascularity and oxygen, thereby retarding collagen synthesis).[5]

a. Compressive techniques
    i. Pressure garments (Fig. 1-7).
    ii. Silastic molds and gel sheets (Fig. 1-8).

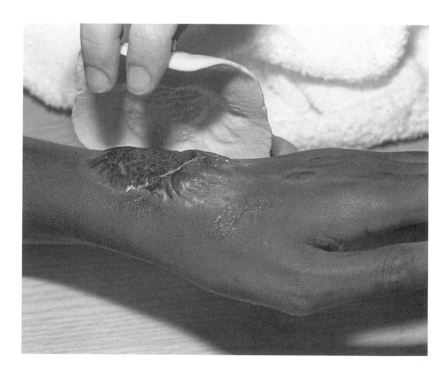

Fig. 1-8. Elastomer mold.

        b. Splinting. (Requires low-load, long duration application of stress for permanent elongation of scar).

        c. AROM and PROM exercise.

        d. Deep friction massage.

        e. Mechanical vibration.

    4. Thermal agents to increase tissue extensibility before stretching and ROM exercise

        a. Superficial heat (paraffin, hot packs, fluidotherapy)

        b. Deep heat (ultrasound)

C. Functional

    1. Exercises and activities to increase strength, endurance, and function in the injured extremity

COMPLICATIONS

I. Infections

II. Wound dehiscence

III. Abnormal scar formation

    A. Hypertrophic

    B. Keloid

EVALUATION TIMELINE

Wound status and type of dressing should be assessed at every treatment, during initial and discharge evaluations, and each time a progress evaluation is indicated for that patient, up until the wound is healed. After wound closure, description of scar and resulting limitations of motion, strength, and function should be noted.

REFERENCES

1. Feedar JA, Kloth LC: Conservative management of chronic wounds. p. 135. In Kloth LC, McCulloch JM, Feedar JA (eds): Wound Healing: Alternatives in Management. FA Davis, Philadelphia, 1990
2. Mullins PT: Use of therapeutic modalities in upper extremity rehabilitation. p. 195. In Hunter JM, Schneider LH, Mackin EJ, Callahan AD (eds): Rehabilitation of the Hand: Surgery and Therapy. 3rd Ed. CV Mosby, Baltimore, 1990
3. Donnell M: Pros and cons of wound care techniques for the upper extremity. Practice Forum. J Hand Ther 3:128, 1991
4. Evans RB: An update on wound management. Hand Clin 7:409, 1991
5. Hardy MA: The biology of scar formation. Phys Ther 69:1014, 1989

SUGGESTED READINGS

Alvarez O, Rozint J, Wiseman D: Moist environment for healing: matching the dressing to the wound. Wounds 1:35, 1989

Arem AJ, Madden JW: Effects of stress on healing wounds: I. intermittent noncyclical tension. J Surg Res 20:93, 1976

Ahn ST, Monafo WW, Mustoe TA: Topical silicone gel: a new treatment for hypertrophic scars. Surgery 106:781, 1989

Brennan SS, Foster ME, Leaper DJ: Antiseptic toxicity in wounds healing by secondary intention. J Hosp Infect 8:263, 1986

Bruster J, Pullium G: Gradient pressure. Am J Occup Ther 37:485, 1983

Bryant W: Clinical Symposia: Wound healing. CIBA Pharmaceutical Co., Summit, 1977

Burkhalter WE: Wound classification and management. p. 167. In Hunter JM, Schneider LH, Mackin EJ, Callahan AD (eds): Rehabilitation of the Hand: Surgery and Therapy. 3rd Ed. CV Mosby, Baltimore, 1990

Carrico T, Merhof A, Cohen I: Biology of wound healing. Surg Clin North Am 64: 721, 1984

Clark JA, Cheng JC, Leung KS, Leung PC: Mechanical characterization of human postburn hypertrophic skin during pressure therapy. J Biomech 20:397, 1987

Cohen K: Can collagen metabolism be controlled: theoretical considerations. J Trauma 25:410, 1985

Cohn GH: Hyperbaric oxygen therapy: promoting healing in difficult cases. Postgrad Med Oxygen Ther 79:89, 1986

Davies D: Scars, hypertrophic scars, and keloids. Br Med J Clin Res 290:1056, 1985

Dow Corning Wright Monograph: Silastic gel sheeting. Arlington, TN, 1989

Groves AR: The problem with scars. Burns 13:S15, 1987

Henning JP, Roskam Y, Van Gemert MJ: Treatment of keloids and hypertrophic scars with an argon laser. Lasers Surg Med 6:72, 1986

Hunt TK (ed): Wound Healing and Wound Infection: Theory and Surgical Practice. Appleton-Century-Crofts, New York, 1980

Hunt TK, Dunphy J: Fundamentals of Wound Management. Appleton-Century-Crofts, East Norwalk, CT, 1979

Hunt TK, Lavan FB: Enhancement of wound healing by growth factors. N Engl J Med 321:111, 1989

Jensen LL, Parshley PF: Postburn scar contractures: histology and effects of pressure treatment. J Burn Care Rehabil 5:119, 1984

Johnson CL: Physical therapists as scar modifiers. Phys Ther 64:1381, 1984

Johnson CL: Wound healing and scar formation. Top Acute Care Trauma Rehabil 1:1, 1987

Kanzler MH, Gorsulowsky DC, Swanson NA: Basic mechanisms in the healing cutaneous wound. J Dermatol Surg Oncol 12:1156, 1986

Kloth LC, Feedar JA: Acceleration of wound healing with high voltage, monophasic, pulsed current. Phys Ther 68:503, 1988

Kloth LC, McCulloch JM, Feedar JA: Wound Healing: Alternatives in Management. FA Davis, Philadelphia, 1990

Lawrence JC: The aetiology of scars. Burns 13:S3, 1987

Linares HA, Kischer CA, Dobrkovsky M, Larson DL: On the origin of the hypertrophic scar. J Trauma 13:70, 1973

Madden JW: Wound healing: the biological basis of hand surgery. p. 181. In Hunter JM, Schneider LH, Mackin EJ, Callahan AD (eds): Rehabilitation of the Hand: Surgery and Therapy. 3rd Ed. CV Mosby, Baltimore, 1990

Malick MH, Carr JA: Flexible elastomer molds in burn scar control. Am J Occup Ther 34:603, 1980

Michlovitz SL: Thermal Agents in Rehabilitation. 2nd Ed. FA Davis, Philadelphia, 1990

Nicolai JP, Bronkhorst FB, Smale CE: A protocol for the treatment of hypertrophic scars and keloids. Aesth Plast Surg 11:29, 1987

Noe JM: Wound Care. 2nd Ed. Chesebrough-Pond's Inc., Greenwich, 1985

Noe JM: Dressing the acutely injured hand. p. 241. In Wolfort FG (ed): Acute Hand Injuries: A Multispecialty Approach. Little, Brown, Boston, 1980

Noe JM, Keller M: Can stitches get wet? Plast Reconstr Surg 81.82, 1988

Peacock EE: Wound Repair. 3rd Ed. WB Saunders, Philadelphia, 1984

Peacock EE, Madden JW, Trier WC: Biologic basis for the treatment of keloids and hypertrophic scars. S Med J 63:755, 1970

Perkins K, Davey RB, Wallis K: Current materials and techniques used in a burn scar management programme. Burns 13:406, 1987

Pollack SV: Wound healing: a review. J Dermatol Surg Oncol 5:389, 1979

Quinn KJ: Silicone gel in scar treatment. Burns 13:S33, 1987

Quinn KJ, Evans JH, Courtney JM et al: Non-pressure treatment of hypertrophic scars. Burns 12:102, 1985

Reid W: Hypertrophic scarring and pressure therapy. Burns 13:S29, 1987

Rodeheaver G, Bellamy W, Kody M et al: Bactericidal activity and toxicity of iodine-containing solutions in wounds. Arch Surg 117:181, 1982

Rose MP, Deitch EA: The clinical use of a tubular compression bandage, Tubigrip, for burn-scar therapy: a critical analysis. Burns 12:58, 1985

Ross R: Wound healing. Sci Am 220:40, 1969

Rudolph R: Wide spread scars, hypertrophic scars, and keloids. Clin Plast Surg 14:253, 1987

Smith KL: Wound care for the hand patient. p. 172. In Hunter JM, Schneider LH, Mackin EJ, Callahan AD (eds): Rehabilitation of the Hand: Surgery and Therapy. 3rd Ed. CV Mosby, Baltimore, 1990

Surveyer JA, Cloughtery DM: Burn scars: fighting the effects. Am J Nurs 83:746, 1983

Weeks P, Wray C: Hand Management: A Biological Approach. CV Mosby, St. Louis, 1973

Wessling N, Ehleben CM, Chapman V et al: Evidence that use of a silicone gel sheet increases range of motion over burn wound contractures. J Burn Care Rehabil 6:503, 1985

Westaby S (ed): Wound Care. CV Mosby, St. Louis, 1986

Appendix 1-1

WOUND HEALING PHASE TIMETABLE

I. Epithelialization (begins within a few hours after wounding).
   A. Regeneration of epithelial layer through four stages: mobilization, migration, proliferation, and differentiation of epithelial cells.
   B. Covers exposed dermis.
   C. May be complete in 6 to 48 hours after suturing (longer in wound healing by secondary intention).

II. Inflammatory (substrate or lag phase: from wounding to 3 to 5 days)
   A. Vascular response (5 to 10 minutes of vasoconstriction followed by vasodilation)
   B. Phagocytosis (neutrophils and macrophages rid wound of bacteria and foreign debris)

III. Fibroplasia (latent phase: days 4 to 5 to days 14 to 28
   A. Fibroblasts enter wound and begin synthesizing collagen (scar tissue).
   B. Tensile strength increases with deposition of collagen.
   C. Angiogenesis (neovascularization): capillary budding begins, to form new blood vessels.
   D. Formation of granulation tissue (new collagen and new capillaries, red in appearance).

IV. Scar maturation or remodeling (days 14 to 28 up to several years)
   A. Strength increases through gradual intramolecular and intermolecular cross linking of collagen molecules.
   B. Changes occur in form, bulk, and architecture of collagen (i.e., ongoing collagen synthesis versus lysis cycle; more organized orientation of collagen fibers with applied stress).
   C. Appearance of scar will change from red and raised to a more pale and flat scar as maturation occurs.

V. Contraction (days 4 to 5 up to day 21)
   A. Movement of wound margins toward center of wound defect.
   B. Myofibroblasts (a modified fibroblast) thought to be responsible for wound contraction.

Appendix 1-2

WOUND HEALING PROCESS

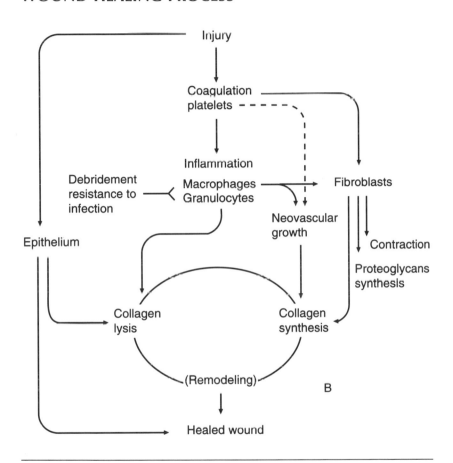

(From Levenson S, Seifter E, Van Winkle W: Nutrition. p. 286. In Hunt TK, Dunphy J (eds): Fundamentals of Wound Management. Appleton-Century-Crofts, East Norwalk, CT, 1979, with permission.)

Skin Grafts and Flaps

2

Mallory S. Anthony

Wounds with significant tissue loss often require skin grafts or flaps for adequate wound closure. In the hand, replacement of soft tissue warrants special attention since maximum functional outcome is imperative. Dorsal skin must be thinner, more elastic, loose enough not to restrict flexion, and serve as a barrier to cover tendons and joints.[1] Volar skin must be thicker and tougher (to withstand pressure and friction caused by grasp and pinch), be loose and elastic enough to allow motion, and retain its function of sensibility.[1]

Firm "take" of a skin graft requires good recipient bed vascularity, free from increased levels of bacteria and devitalized tissue. After application of a skin graft, the graft first survives by transudate from the wound (plasmatic circulation).[1] Later, the ingrowth of capillary buds into the skin graft from the wound bed provides the necessary vascularity. Optimal beds for skin grafts include muscle and fascia. Suboptimal beds include denuded bone or tendon.

A split-thickness skin graft (STSG) is generally obtained from the thigh, buttock, or abdomen. Advantages of these skin grafts include: (1) more suitable on large and contaminated wounds, (2) take more readily, (3) less prone to infection, and (4) large supply of donor sites. One major disadvantage is its increased tendency to contract during healing.

A full-thickness skin graft (FTSG) is generally obtained from the hypothenar eminence, medial aspect of the arm, or groin. Advantages of these skin grafts include: (1) increased durability, (2) afford better protection, (3) establish better sensibility, (4) contain more epidermal appendages, (5) contract less than STSGs, (6) provide increased cosmesis and color match, and (7) more suitable for small, clean wounds (Fig. 2-1).

Skin flaps are needed for soft tissue coverage when the recipient bed provides poor vascularity. A skin flap consists of dermis and subcutaneous tissue, elevated from its underlying bed, and maintains its vascularity

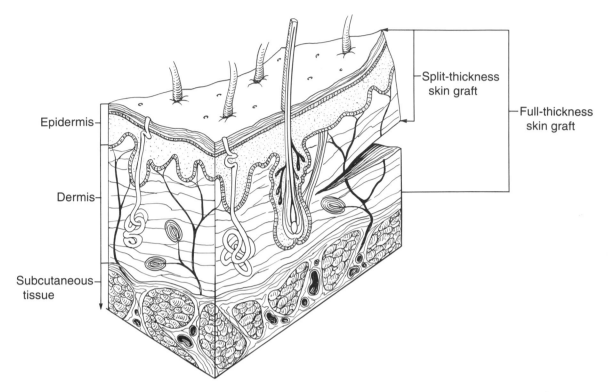

Epidermis

Dermis

Subcutaneous tissue

Split-thickness skin graft

Full-thickness skin graft

Fig. 2-1. Split- and full-thickness skin grafts.

through its base (pedicle). This pedicle consists of the full thickness of the dermis and subcutaneous tissues, and contains the subdermal vascular plexus.[2] Since random skin flaps are dependent for their blood supply on the subdermal plexus, they can be raised at any site of the body or in any direction.[2] There are, however, limitations in their dimensions (i.e., the length should not exceed the width of the pedicle). In the case of the axial flap, there are identifiable, cutaneous vessels in the pedicle that provide a better blood supply, and have less tendency toward venous engorgement.[2]

The edges of all these skin flaps initially depend upon nutrition by perfusion through microcirculation, before neovascularization (capillary budding) occurs and sufficient blood supply has grown across into the flap from the surrounding tissues. Approximately 3 weeks is required before healing is sufficient to allow pedicle division.

Pedicle flaps can provide sufficient tissue coverage in all but the most massive defects.[3] However, the hand must be dependent during attachment, resulting in prolonged immobilization; these flaps require a minimum of two operative procedures; the blood supply upon which the pedicle flap is initially dependent is cut at the time of detachment, making the flap dependent upon peripheral vascularity (less dependable and ro-

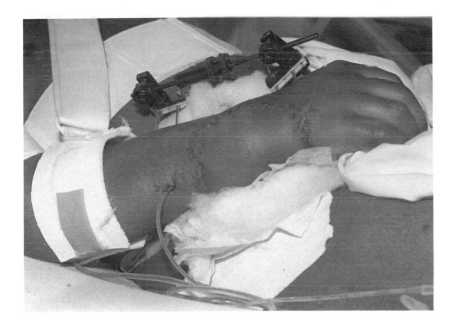

Fig. 2-2. Pedicle flap from groin for soft tissue defect. External fixator for treatment of distal forearm fracture.

bust); and the flap may be avulsed by a very young or incompetent patient (Fig. 2-2).

A free flap provides immediate vascularity and is transferred by dividing its vascular pedicle and resuturing the pedicle to recipient vessels in the recipient site. Vein grafts are sometimes necessary if the vascular pedicle is stretched at the repair site. Free flaps offer many advantages over the pedicle flap: (1) the recipient limb is mobile and free of prolonged attachment to the donor, permitting elevation and early mobilization; (2) free flaps frequently require only one operative procedure; (3) they bring their own blood supply, increasing the potential for healing, especially in a poorly vascularized and scarred bed; and (4) they can be cut to fit the defect with incomparable precision (almost limitless choice of size and thickness).[3]

Independent of the type of soft tissue coverage chosen for the patient, our role is to promote wound healing, decrease edema, provide effective scar management, and help restore optimal range of motion (ROM) and function for these patients.

DEFINITIONS

I. Graft: a portion of tissue, such as skin, periosteum bone, or fascia that is severed free and transferred to correct a defect in the body. A graft may consist of skin only (skin graft) or it may be a composite of tissues such as skin, muscle, or bone (composite graft).[4]

II. Flap: a portion of tissue *partly* severed from its place of origin to correct a defect in the body. A flap may also consist of skin only

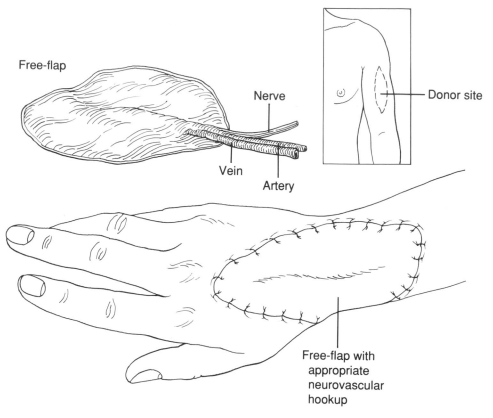

Fig. 2-3. Various flaps may be considered for coverage.

(including its subdermal plexus of vessels), or it may be a composite of tissues such as skin, muscle, or bone (composite flap).[4] A flap contains its own vascular supply (Fig. 2-3).

III. Types of tissue transfers
  A. Free tissue transfers
    1. STSG: a free graft of skin that includes the epidermis and part of the dermis. (May be meshed where moderate serous drainage is expected or when recipient bed is suboptimal for vascularity.)
    2. FTSG: a free graft of skin that includes the whole thickness of epidermis and dermis. Contains dermal appendages and nerve endings, with the exception of subcutaneous sweat glands and some Pacinian corpuscles.
    3. Free vascularized tissue transfer: a composite flap with its vascular pedicle completely cut and transferred to the recipient site for immediate microvascular anastomoses (e.g., free groin flap, free latissimus flap).
  B. Pedicled flaps (require later detachment)
    1. Random: designed to fit the recipient defect without attention

to specific nutrient vessels in the pedicle.[4] There is no anatomically recognized arterial or venous system and it receives its blood supply from the dermal–subdermal plexus (e.g., Z-plasty, V–Y advancement, rotation flap, transposition flap).
    2. Axial: designed so that the pedicle has within it identifiable, direct, cutaneous vascular elements.[4]
        a. Cutaneous: axial flaps whose vessels supply skin alone and proceed directly to it (e.g., groin flap).
        b. Fasciocutaneous: axial flaps whose vessels first supply fascia (e.g., lateral arm flap).
        c. Myocutaneous or musculocutaneous: axial flaps whose vessels first supply muscle (e.g., latissimus dorsi flap).
        d. Island flap: an axial flap whose pedicle has been reduced to the point that it consists only of nutrient blood vessels with or without nerves (e.g., neurovascular digital island flap).
IV. Location of grafts/flaps
    A. Local (from skin adjacent to the defect); for example, transposition (Z-plasty), advancement (V–Y advancement), or rotation (Fillet flap).
    B. Regional (from elsewhere on the limb); for example, lateral arm flap, cross-finger flap, or thenar flap.
    C. Distant (from other parts of the body); for example, abdominal or groin flap.

SURGICAL PURPOSE

To provide wound coverage of open areas to protect underlying structures. Each graft type has a very specific reason for being used, and each has well-defined risk–benefit ratios.

TREATMENT GOALS

I. Provide adequate wound care and promote wound healing of graft, flap, and/or donor site.
II. Restore active ROM ((AROM) and passive ROM (PROM) in affected areas underlying flaps/grafts.
III. Maintain full ROM of all uninvolved joints.
IV. Return to previous level of function.

INDICATIONS FOR TISSUE COVERAGE

I. Split-thickness and full-thickness grafts are used to replace skin in areas where adequate subcutaneous tissues remain to protect underlying structures, and where adequate circulation is available.

II. Flaps are indicated in wounds where there is bone devoid of periosteum, tendon devoid of paratenon, cartilage devoid of perichondrium, or exposed vital structures.

PRECAUTIONS FOR THERAPY

I. Decreased graft/flap viability
   A. Infection (cardinal signs: warmth, redness, pain, and edema)
   B. Mechanical problems: establishment of barrier between bed and graft (e.g., hematoma)
   C. Inadequate preparation of recipient bed
   D. Inadequate surgical technique
II. Damage and repair to deep vital structures
III. Extreme pain
IV. Severe edema

THERAPY

I. Preoperative management
   A. Provide sterile whirlpool, dressing changes, and debridement of recipient wound area, if indicated, in preparation for tissue coverage.
   B. Patient education to prepare patient for pedicle or free flap. This may include instruction in one-handed techniques and information regarding the type of clothing that will best accommodate the arm while it is attached, as in the case of a groin flap.
   C. Maximize ROM and increase strength in muscle to be transferred for planned functional muscle flap (nonemergency basis).
II. Postoperative evaluation
   A. Please refer to wound management evaluation, Chapter 1.
   B. Graft/flap viability assessment (general guidelines).[5]
      1. Observe color
         a. Random pattern flap
            i. *Pink*: healthy
            ii. *Pale* with faint *blue/grey tinge*: inadequate arterial supply
            iii. *Angry red* first, then progressively *purple red* and *purple blue*: inadequate venous supply
         b. Axial pattern flap
            i. *Very pale pink*: healthy
            ii. *Waxy pallor* (white tinged with yellow or brown): vascular compromise
         c. Free flaps
            i. *Pink*: healthy
            ii. *White* or *mottled appearance*: arterial problems
            iii. *Dusky blue*: venous problems

    2. Observe refill after blanching by fingertip pressure or by running a blunt point across flap.
       a. Slow refill with pale flap: arterial insufficiency
       b. Rapid refill with bluish flap: venous insufficiency (e.g, kinking of pedicle)
    3. Temperature of flap
       Marked difference (decrease) in temperature between flap and tissue adjacent to flap may indicate impaired blood flow.
    4. Monitor pulsatile flow within the flap.

III. Postoperative management (skin grafts).[1,6]
  A. Grafts immobilized and protected 4 to 5 days for STSG and 5 to 7 days for FTSG.
  B. 5 to 7 days postoperatively may begin daily dressing changes with nonadherent gauze.

    *Please note: loss of a graft is usually the result of shear forces, fluid accumulation under graft, tension, or purulence. Care must be taken during dressing changes not to rub the healing graft.

  C. Seventh postoperative day, begin *gentle* ROM exercises (under supervision of therapist only). May want to exercise without dressing in place to avoid a shearing force on the wound.
  D. Elevation to decrease edema (no compressive wraps until at least 2 weeks postoperatively, and only after consulting the treating physician).
  E. 1 week postoperatively, sterile whirlpool and wound care to clean wound and stimulate local circulation.
  F. 10 to 14 days: gentle application of topical lubricant to healed areas, as graft sites are dry due to lack of secondary protective skin structures.
  G. 2 weeks postoperatively, pressure garments and compressive wraps may be used over a well-vascularized graft to decrease edema, if shearing forces are avoided, and after consulting treating physician.
  H. 3 to 4 weeks postoperatively: gentle massage and scar-softening modalities.
  I. Splinting
    1. Early/protective: to immobilize joints in functional position, eliminate tension on repaired structures, and protect the healing graft.
    2. Late (6 weeks): to apply stress to scar and increase ROM.
  J. Continue ROM exercises and add activities to increase strength, endurance, and function.
  K. Monitor return of sensation.
  L. Caution patients against exposure of either graft donor or recipient sites to the sun for at least 6 months.

IV. Postoperative management (flaps)[6]
  A. Pedicle (axial)
    1. Left attached 2 to 4 weeks (to allow new vascular ingrowth to the flap from the recipient bed).

2. Use gauze pads in areas where maceration is a problem.
3. String wrapping or coban to free digits and retrograde massage to decrease edema if no stress is placed on attachment.
4. Maintain ROM in uninvolved joints.
5. After flap detachment.
   a. Promote wound healing.
   b. Decrease edema.
   c. Regain active and passive motion in uninvolved joints.
   d. Re-establish active and passive ROM in affected area.
   e. Scar management.
B. Free tissue transfer.[5,6]
   1. Vascular status is critical in the first few days postoperatively. (Patient is kept warm and should abstain from caffeine and nicotine.)
   2. Elevation to heart level only to decrease edema. Extensive elevation may impair arterial inflow.
   3. 8 to 10 days: flap should be stable.
      a. Wound care for donor and recipient sites. (If wounds are dry and healing well, minimal dressing is required. If not, whirlpool may be initiated once the flap is thought to be stable by treating physician.)
      b. Monitor vascularity: observe color, temperature, and capillary refill time.
      c. Continue elevation for edema control (no compressive wraps until at least third postoperative week, and only with physician approval).
      d. AROM to uninvolved joints.
   4. 2 weeks: AROM of involved joints if vascular status is stable.
   5. 3 to 4 weeks: gentle massage, scar-softening modalities, and compressive wraps if vascular status is stable.
   6. 6 to 8 weeks: splinting and passive ROM exercise as healing permits.
   7. 8 weeks: patient can resume normal daily activities using the hand.
   8. Continue ROM exercises and add activities to increase strength, endurance, and function.
   9. Heavy and stressful activities allowed at 3 months.
   10. Monitor return of sensation.
C. Functional muscle flap (free tissue transfer)[6]
   1. Immobilized for 3 weeks in relaxed position. During this immobilization phase, once vascular stability is achieved (usually by 1 to 2 weeks), and with physician approval, PROM of uninvolved joints may be initiated.
   2. Continue gentle PROM exercises until preoperative ROM is achieved.
   3. As clinical signs of reinnervation are noted (4 to 7 months postoperatively), active–assistive ROM exercises may be initiated.

4. Muscle stimulation, active exercise, and resistive exercise may be added as muscle strengthens.

V. Donor sites
   A. Monitor donor site for development of hypertrophic scar.
   B. Massage with topical lubricant and application of pressure may be initiated for scar management, as wound healing permits.
   C. Be aware of loss of sensibility in donor site and educate patient, if a nerve has been taken for a transfer.

POSTOPERATIVE COMPLICATIONS

I. Loss of graft/flap
   A. Hematoma or seroma
   B. Infection
   C. Vascular compromise
      1. Kinking of pedicle attachment
      2. Compression of arterial supply for free flap
      3. Inadequate preparation of recipient bed
II. Extreme pain
III. Severe edema
IV. Excess scarring due to a long interval between injury and time of coverage

EVALUATION TIMELINE

Graft/flap viability status should be assessed at initial evaluation, and during every treatment session until the graft or flap is well-taken. Joint motion affected by graft/flap should be assessed when changes occur or at least once a month. Mobility and description of scar should be assessed, as well as sensory status, strength, and function during these follow-up evaluations.

REFERENCES

1. Browne EZ: Skin grafts. p. 1805. In Green DP (ed): Operative Hand Surgery. 2nd Ed. Churchill Livingstone, New York, 1988
2. Smith PF: Skin loss and scar contractures. p. 31. In Burke FD, McGrouther DA, Smith PJ (eds): Principles of Hand Surgery. Churchill Livingstone, New York, 1990
3. Lister G: Emergency free flaps. p. 1127. In Green DP (ed): Operative Hand Surgery. 2nd Ed. Churchill Livingstone, New York, 1988
4. Chase RA: Skin and soft tissue. p. 1. In: Atlas of Hand Surgery. Vol. 2 . WB Saunders, Philadelphia, 1984
5. Lister G: Skin flaps. p. 1839. In Green DP (ed): Operative Hand Surgery. 2nd Ed. Churchill Livingstone, New York, 1988
6. Singer DI, Moore JH, Bryon PM: Management of skin grafts and flaps. p. 253.

In Hunter JM, Schneider LH, Mackin EJ, Callahan AD (eds): Rehabilitation of the Hand: Surgery and Therapy. 3rd Ed. CV Mosby, Baltimore, 1990

SUGGESTED READINGS

(Please also refer to wound management suggested readings.)

Beasley RW: Hand Injuries. WB Saunders, Philadelphia, 1981

Brown PW: Open injuries of the hand. p. 1619. In Green DP (ed): Operative Hand Surgery. 2nd Ed. Churchill Livingstone, New York, 1988

Browne EZ: Complications of skin grafts and pedicle flaps. Hand Clin 2:353, 1986

Jabaley ME: Recovery of sensation in flaps and skin grafts. p. 583. In Tubiana R (ed): The Hand. Vol. 1. WB Saunders, Philadelphia, 1981

Ketchum L: Skin and soft tissue coverage of the upper extremity. Hand Clin 4(1), 1985

Lister G: The theory of the transposition flap and its practical application in the hand. Clin Plast Surg 8:115, 1981

Lister G: Injury. p. 1. In: The Hand: Diagnosis and Indications. 2nd Ed. Churchill Livingstone, New York, 1984

Mathes SJ, Alpert BS: Free skin and composite flaps. p. 1151. In Green DP (ed): Operative Hand Surgery. 2nd Ed. Churchill Livingstone, New York, 1988

Michon J: Complex hand injuries: surgical planning. p. 196. In Tubiana R (ed): The Hand. Vol. 2. WB Saunders, Philadelphia, 1985

Morrison WA, Gilbert A: Complications in microsurgery. p. 145. In Tubiana R (ed): The Hand. Vol. 2. WB Saunders, Philadelphia, 1985

Tsuge K, Kanaujia RR, Steichen JB: Comprehensive Atlas of Hand Surgery. Year Book Medical Publishers, Chicago, 1989

Weeks P, Wray C: Wound healing and tissue coverage. p. 3. In: Hand Management: A Biological Approach. CV Mosby, St. Louis, 1973

Wolfort FG: Acute Hand Injuries: A Multispeciality Approach. Little, Brown, Boston, 1980

Appendix 2-1

Type of Soft Tissue Coverage	Vascularity/Take	Donor Site Closure
STSG	3 days	Secondary intention
FTSG	5–7 days	Primary intention
Pedicled flaps	Approximately 3 weeks	Primary closure or skin graft
Free tissue transfer	Immediate	Primary closure or skin graft

STSG, split-thickness skin graft; FTSC, full-thickness skin graft.

Burns

3

Beth Farrell

Hand burns are the most common of all thermal injuries,[1-3] and if left untreated, can result in severe deformities and loss of function. The following protocol serves as a guideline for treatment of thermal injuries to the hand/upper extremity.

Thermal injuries are categorized according to the level of underlying destruction. Partial-thickness burns are termed "superficial" when there is destruction of the epidermis and possibly portions of the dermis.[4] This type of burn is very painful, but does not require skin grafting.[4] In full-thickness burns, the entire epidermal and dermal layers have been destroyed.[4] Thus, skin grafting is necessary to achieve joint motion and underlying tendon gliding[2,4,5] (Fig. 3-1).

Therapeutic intervention of the burned upper extremity requires a therapist trained specifically in the following areas: wound/graft care, splinting to prevent deformities/contractures, edema control, scar management, and pain control.

Immediately postoperatively, splinting is required to position the hand in an anti-deformity position. Active range of motion (AROM) exercises are initiated about 1 week postoperatively and the patient is instructed to use the hand for light activities as tolerated. Pain is controlled by transcutaneous electrical nerve stimulation (TENS) or a microdyne. Hypertrophic scarring can result in joint contractures and tendon adherence; therefore, it is important to initiate scar management once tissues are healed.

Compressive garments are often necessary for minimizing hypertrophic scarring[2,4,5] (Fig. 3-2). Pressure garments also aid in the reduction of edema. Elevation of the extremity, which is initiated immediately postoperatively and as needed thereafter, is also extremely important in controlling edema.

In summary, therapeutic intervention is extremely important when treating a burned hand/upper extremity for several reasons: to prevent

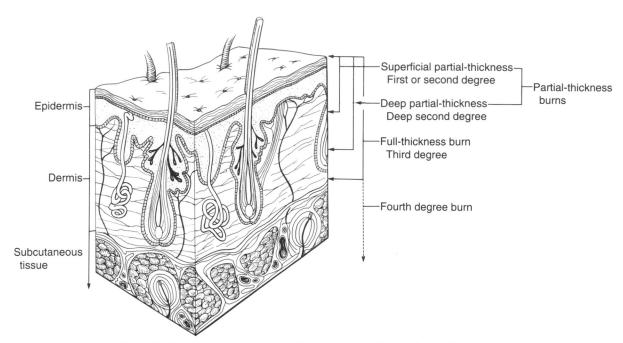

Fig. 3-1. Categorization of thermal injuries according to level of injury.

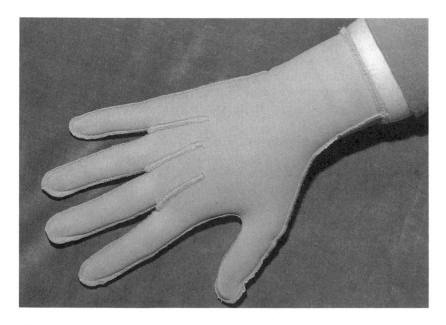

Fig. 3-2. Compressive garments are used to minimize hypertrophic scarring.

potential deformities, minimize complications, and return patients to their previous level of functioning.

DEFINITION

Injuries to soft tissues caused by contact with dry heat (e.g., fire), moist heat (e.g., steam or hot liquid), chemicals, electricity, friction, or radiant energy.[6]

I. Partial-thickness burns[4]
   A. Superficial partial-thickness: first or second degree burn (i.e., destruction of epidermis and possibly portions of upper dermal layers). Appears red, bright pink, blistered, wet, and soft. Painful. No grafting necessary for healing.
   B. Deep partial-thickness: deep second degree burn. Destruction of epidermis and greater portion of dermal layer (hair follicles, sweat glands). Appears red or white, wet, soft, elastic. Sensation may be diminished. Potential conversion to full thickness burn.
II. Full-thickness burn[2,4]
   Third degree burn. Destruction of entire epidermis and dermal layers (hair follicles, nerve endings, sweat glands). Requires skin grafting. Appears white or tan, waxy, dry, leathery, nonelastic.
III. Fourth degree burn
   Deep soft tissue damage to fat, muscle, and bone
IV. Electrical Burn[4]
   Thrombosed blood vessels, destruction of nerves along pathway, possible fractures, dislocations. Requires surgical excision of necrotic tissue. Possible amputation.

TREATMENT AND SURGICAL PURPOSE

To prevent deformity where burns have occurred and to restore parts where damaged or lost. Of greatest concern is the loss of skin and joint mobility in critical areas such as with the wrist and digits. Proper splinting to prevent deformity and maintain function is essential. Skin resurfacing is frequently required to achieve joint motion and underlying tendon gliding. Resurfacing where scar contractures exist that cause deformity will also necessitate skin grafting.

TREATMENT GOALS

I. Maximize functional recovery through prevention of the following.
   A. Contractures
   B. Infection
   C. Edema

D. Muscle disuse atrophy
E. Tendon adherence
F. Capsular shortening
II. Control pain.
III. Achieve wound closure by protecting regenerating epithelial cells.[1]

INDICATIONS FOR SURGERY

I. Tangential excision/grafting: Indicated for deep partial-thickness burns.
II. Full-thickness excision: indicated for full-thickness burns.
III. Thermal burn: may require an escharotomy.
IV. Electrical burn: may require fasciotomy.[3]

POSTOPERATIVE INDICATIONS/PRECAUTIONS FOR THERAPY

I. Contraindications for open wounds
   A. Excessive heat on burn wound (will cause sloughing).
   B. Serial casting.
   C. Overstretching and vigorous exercise.[2,4,5,7]
   D. Occlusive dressing (interferes with evaluation of perfusion).[3]
   E. Splinting straps may interfere with circulation. Gauze wraps may be an alternative.
   F. Pressure areas caused by splinting may increase severity of burn.[5]
   G. Discontinue range of motion (ROM) to exposed joints or tendons.[4]
   H. Discontinue ROM if patient complains of deep joint pain.
   I. Cellulitis.[4]
II. Contraindications during entire rehabilitation program
   A. Patient should avoid the following
      1. Strong sunlight.
      2. Rubbing skin.
      3. Contact with heat, radiators.
      4. Cold weather: patient should wear gloves.
      5. Vascular insufficiency may lead to compartment syndrome if not treated.[1]

POSTOPERATIVE THERAPY

I. See graft care guidelines for specific management.
II. See wound care guidelines for specifics on management of wounds.
III. Superficial partial-thickness burns
   A. First 48 hours: keep hand elevated.[3,5] Sterile whirlpool. See physician regarding debridement approach. Dress with nonadherent dressing. Begin gentle AROM and passive range of motion

(PROM) to pain tolerance. Microdyne (HVPC) may be indicated to control edema and pain.[1] Splinting as indicated.

   B. 2 days to healing of wounds: encourage independence in activities of daily living (ADL); full mobility.[2,4,7]

IV. Deep partial-thickness burns if *not grafted*

   A. Up to 72 hours postoperative: keep hand elevated.[3,5] Irrigate wound with saline. Remove debris. Dress with nonadherent dressing. Edema control as indicated. Pain control as indicated. Begin gentle AROM. AROM exercise should be performed every hour.[1]

      1. Lumbrical plus position

      2. Abduction/adduction of fingers

For dorsal hand burn, hook and fist exercises may be initiated as soon as viability of the extensor tendons is known.[1] Splint in intrinsic-plus position; that is, wrist 20 degrees to 30 degrees extension, metacarpophalangeal (MCP) joints: 70 degrees flexion; interphalangeal (IP) joints full extension; thumb abducted and extended[1,4] (Fig. 3-3).

   B. Once edema has decreased: splint only at night and during rest periods. Begin PROM to tolerance. Provide patient with sponge to encourage increased ROM. Encourage use of hand for light activities.

   C. Once wound has healed: begin gradual strengthening as tolerated.

V. Full-thickness burn: excision/grafting or deep partial-thickness burn

   A. Immediately postoperative: Hand is elevated.[3,5] Splint in intrinsic plus position unless the dorsal surface of the hand and fingers are

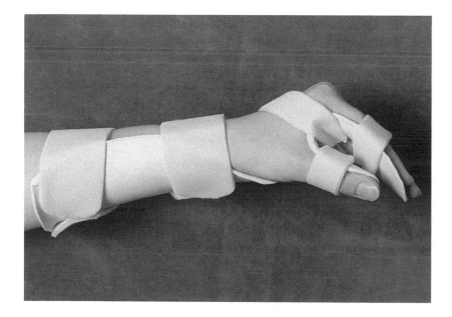

Fig. 3-3. Splint design to be used with dorsal hand burns.

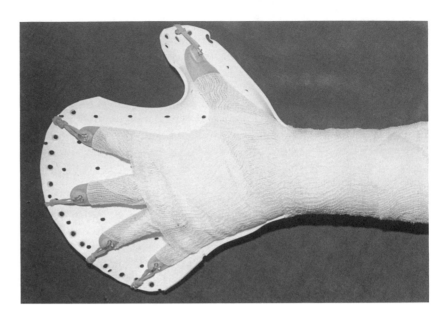

Fig. 3-4. Splint for dorsal hand and finger grafts.

grafted; then splint with fingers in abduction, and consider use of fingernail hooks for proper positioning and tension (Fig. 3-4).

B. 72 hours postoperative: First dressing change.[4] Consult with patient's physician regarding appropriate type of dressing. Splint at all times. Continue to keep hand elevated. Pain control as indicated.

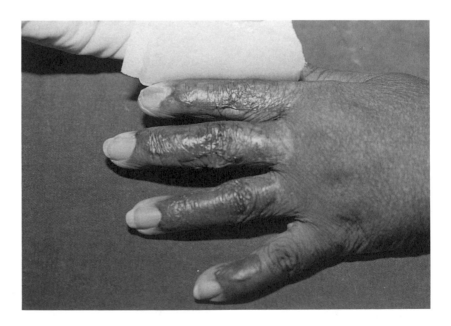

Fig. 3-5. Gel sheet application for scar management.

C. 5 to 7 days: Daily dressing changes. Take off splint to exercise. Begin gentle AROM exercises as described in IV.A.[4,5] Encourage light ADL.[4] Begin sterile whirlpool as soon as edema has minimized. Discontinue whirlpool if edema increases with its use.

D. Over 7 days: Decrease splinting time unless patient begins to develop deformities. Begin PROM to tolerance (stretching of thumb and web space).[4] Encourage use of hand for all self-care activities.

E. Once tissue is healed: Begin friction massage. Begin retrograde massage if needed. Apply elastomer molds or gel sheets to patient's scars (Fig. 3-5). If needed, order compressive burn garments (may use elastomer inserts under compressive garment).[2] Begin occupational training as soon as edema is minimal and patient presents with a good grip. Keep in mind that contractures sometimes do not develop until 2 to 3 weeks postoperatively. Patient should continue to see his/her therapist for splinting and elastomer adjustments as needed.

POSTOPERATIVE COMPLICATIONS

I. Infection
II. Contractures
III. Associated joint disorders (stiff elbow, shoulder)
IV. Fractures under the burn wound
V. Osteomyelitis
VI. Electrically induced heart arrhythmias (electrical burns only)
VII. Pain
VIII. Vascular insufficiency (primarily during the first 72 hours)
IX. Skin maceration (especially when wearing compressive garments)
X. Poor hygiene (especially when wearing compressive garments, elastomer molds, etc.)

EVALUATION TIMELINE

I. ROM
   A. Superficial partial-thickness burns: up to 72 hours postoperatively
   B. Deep partial-thickness burns *not grafted*: up to 72 hours postoperatively
II. Sensory
   For all burns: evaluate as soon as wounds have healed.
III. Strengthening
   For all burns: evaluate as soon as all wounds have healed, edema is minimized, and patient presents with a good grip.

REFERENCES

1. Howell JW: Management of the acutely burned hand for the non-specialized clinician. J Phys Ther 69(12):1077, 1989
2. Hopkins HL, Smith HD: Willard and Spackman's Occupational Therapy. 6th Ed. JB Lippincott, Philadelphia, 1983
3. Salisbury RE, Dingeldein GP: The burned hand and upper extremity. p. 1523. In Green DP (ed): Operative Hand Surgery. 2nd Ed. Vol. 2. Churchill Livingstone, New York, 1988
4. Malick M, Carr J: Manual on Management of the Burned Patient. Harmanville Rehabilitation Center, Pittsburgh, 1982
5. Ostergren G: Burn care. p. 103. In Ziegler EM (ed): Current Concepts in Orthotics: A Diagnosis and Related Approach to Splinting. Roylan Medical Products, Chicago, 1984
6. Dorland's Illustrated Medical Dictionary. 27th Ed. WB Saunders, Philadelphia, 1988
7. Puddicombe BE, Nardone MA: Rehabilitation of the burned hand. p. 281. In Grossman JA (ed): Hand Clinics: Burns of the Upper Extremity. Vol. 6. No. 2. WB Saunders, Philadelphia, 1990

SUGGESTED READINGS

Fisher SV, Helm PA: Comprehensive Rehabilitation of Burns. Williams & Wilkins, Baltimore, 1982
Groencvett F, Kreis W: Burns of the hand. Neth J Surg 6:167, 1985
Habal MB: The burned hand: a planned treatment program. J Trauma 18:587, 1978
Levine NS, Buchanan T: The care of burned upper extremities. p. 107. In Ruberg RL (ed): Clinics in Plastic Surgery: Advances in Burn Care. Vol. 13. No. 1. WB Saunders, Philadelphia, 1988

Dupuytren's Disease

4

Dale Eckhaus

Dupuytren's disease is often cited as being of genetic origin.[1,2] The disease primarily affects individuals of Northern European descent.[1-3] It is often associated with other conditions such as chronic alcoholism, epilepsy, diabetes mellitus, and chronic pulmonary disease.[1-4] The disease onset is usually in the fifth to seventh decade of life.[3] Men are more often affected than women.[1,2] In most instances the ulnar side of the hand is affected.[2,5] The disease can have a slow or rapid progression.[2]

Individuals may sometimes exhibit a Dupuytren's diathesis. In those instances, there is a strong family history, the disease begins at an early age, and there is evidence of fibromatosis in areas other than the volar surface of the hand.[3]

The disease is an active cellular process in the fascia of the hand.[1,3,6] It often presents initially as a nodule in the pretendinous bands of the ring and little fingers.[2,3,5] This is followed by the appearance of tendonlike cords, which are due to the pathologic change in normal fascia.[3,6] The thickening and shortening of the fascia causes contracture.[2]

Nonoperative treatment has been ineffective. Attempts to use splints, steroid injections, and vitamin E have not been helpful.[3,7]

Surgery is indicated when the metacarpophalangeal (MCP) joint contracts to 30 degrees, as this deformity becomes a functional problem. Some surgeons feel that any amount of proximal interphalangeal (PIP) joint contracture warrants surgery. Others feel that 15 degrees or greater is an indication for surgery.[1,3,6] A contracture of a PIP joint is more of a concern than an MCP joint contracture due to their differences in capsular ligament structure.[5]

Many methods of surgical treatment have been reported. No one method has been established.[3] Postoperative management also varies. A common goal to the various methods is to promote wound healing, which minimizes scar and maximizes scar mobility.

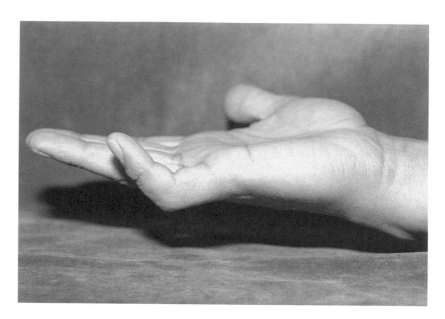

Fig. 4-1. Preoperative positioning of a hand with Dupuytren's disease.

DEFINITION

Disease of fascia of palm and digits (Figs. 4-1 and 4-2).

SURGICAL PURPOSE

Dupuytren's contractures frequently interfere with normal hand function. The deformities are caused by abnormal thickening and contracture of the palmar fascia and its extensions. Surgery is the only method of correcting the problem. The surgical release of the contracture can be

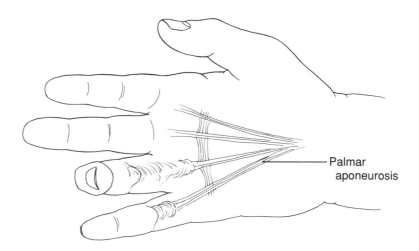

Palmar
aponeurosis

Fig. 4-2. Dupuytren's disease affects the fascia of the hand.

made through varied skin incisions. Neurovascular and tendon elements are frequently in close proximity with the diseased tissues and are therefore vulnerable to injury. Recurrences of the contractures can occur. Some surgeons employ the use of skin grafts to reduce the chances of recurrence. Postoperative hand therapy is an important adjunct to the care of this disease.

TREATMENT GOALS

I. Maintain range of motion (ROM) of uninvolved joints and digits.
II. Control postoperative edema.
III. Promote wound healing especially in open palm techniques.
IV. Improve active ROM (AROM) and passive ROM (PROM) for both extension and flexion.
V. Control and guide scar formation.

NONOPERATIVE INDICATIONS/PRECAUTIONS FOR THERAPY

Nonoperative treatment, including splinting, has not been found to be effective.

POSTOPERATIVE INDICATIONS/PRECAUTIONS FOR THERAPY

I. Indications
    Following surgery of the diseased fascia
II. Precautions
    A. Intraoperative complications involving the neurovascular bundles
    B. Concomitant surgical procedures such as capsulectomy
    C. Skin grafts

POSTOPERATIVE THERAPY

I. During first week, postoperative dressing and splint are replaced with a thin, nonadhesive dressing and either a volar or dorsal removable thermoplastic extension splint. Splints are used periodically during the day and worn throughout the night while sleeping (Fig. 4-3).
II. Whirlpool with extremity positioned horizontally, is utilized early in treatment with an open palm technique or open wounds that result from complications of surgical incisions or grafts.
III. Wound care treatment is employed with appropriate wounds, especially the open techniques.

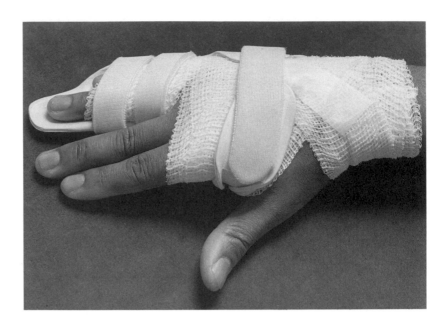

Fig. 4-3. Postoperative thermo-plastic extension splint.

IV. Edema control methods are instituted.
 V. Active, active assisted, and passive range of motion exercises are initiated with first treatment session. Delay or special care in motion may be necessitated by grafts.
VI. Scar management techniques including molded materials are used

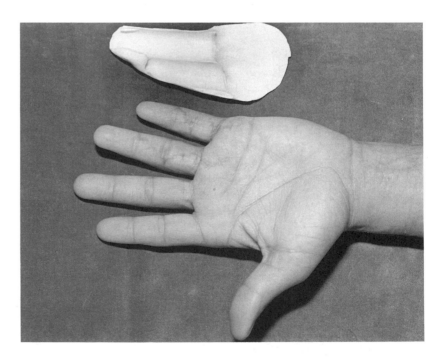

Fig. 4-4. Molded materials are used for scar management.

when wounds are closed and sometimes over nonadherent dressings (Fig. 4-4).

VII. Light activities of daily living (ADL) are permitted in early postoperative phase.

VIII. Light strengthening exercises, progressing to heavier resistance, is introduced once wounds are healed, edema is controlled, and pressure to area is well tolerated.

IX. Splints are adjusted and various types are utilized to achieve full extension and flexion.

X. Splints with scar molds are used for up to 6 months or more.

POSTOPERATIVE COMPLICATIONS

I. Hematoma
II. Edema
III. Skin necrosis
IV. Infection
V. Stiffness
VI. Pain
VII. Reflex sympathetic dystrophy (RSD)
VIII. Recurrence of disease

EVALUATION TIMELINE

I. Initial evaluation of first postoperative visit
   A. Assess the following
      1. Wound and skin condition
      2. Edema
      3. Pain
      4. Sensibility
      5. AROM and PROM
      6. Management of ADL
II. Re-evaluation at 4-week intervals
   Assess strength when wounds are closed and palmar surface can tolerate pressure.

REFERENCES

1. McFarlane RM, Albion U: Dupuytren's disease. p. 867 In Hunter JM, Schneider LH, Mackin EJ, Callahan AD (eds): Rehabilitation of the Hand. 3rd Ed. CV Mosby, St. Louis, 1990

2. Dupuytren's contracture. p. 269. In Schumacher HR, Klippel JF, Robinson DR (eds): Primer on Rheumatic Diseases. 9th Ed. Arthritis Foundation, Atlanta, 1988

3. Hill NA, Hurst LC: Dupuytren's contracture. p. 349. In Doyle JR: Landmark

Advances in Hand Surgery. In Peterson BL (ed): Hand Clinics. Vol. 5. WB Saunders, Philadelphia, 1989

4. Hueston JT: Dupuytren's contracture. p. 797. In Flynn JE (ed): Hand Surgery. 3rd Ed. Williams & Wilkins, Baltimore, 1982

5. Lamb DW, Kuczynski K: Dupuytren's disease. p. 635. In Lamb DW, Hooper G, Kuczynski K (eds): The Practice of Hand Surgery. 2nd Ed. Blackwell Scientific Publications, Oxford, 1989

6. McFarlane RM: Dupuytren's contracture. p. 553. In Green DP (ed): Operative Hand Surgery. 2nd Ed. Churchill Livingstone, New York, 1988

7. Abbott K, Denny J, Burke FD, McGauther DA: A review to attitudes to splintage in Dupuytren's contracture. J Hand Surg (Br) 12:326, 1987

SUGGESTED READINGS

Colville J: Dupuytren's contracture—the role of fasciotomy. The Hand 15:162, 1983

Fietti VG, Mackin EJ: Open palm technique in Dupuytren's disease. p. 873. In Hunter JM, Schneider LH, Mackin EJ, Callahan AD (eds): Rehabilitation of the Hand. 3rd Ed. CV Mosby, St. Louis, 1990

Jain AS, Mitchell C, Carus DA: A simple, inexpensive, post-operative management regime following surgery for Dupuytren's contracture. J Hand Surg (Br) 13:259, 1988

McCash CR: The open palm technique in Dupuytren's contracture. Br J Plast Surg 17:271, 1964

McFarlane RM, McGauther DA, Flint M: Dupuytren's disease. In: The Hand and Upper Limb. Vol. 5. Churchill Livingstone, New York, 1990

Sampson SP, Badalamente MA, Hurst LC et al: The use of a passive motion machine in the postoperative rehabilitation of Dupuytren's disease. J Hand Surg 17A:333, 1992

Seuffer AE, Hueston JT: Dupuytren's contracture. In Mitchell MM (ed): Hand Clinics. Vol. 7. WB Saunders, Philadelphia, 1991

Upper Extremity Vessel Repair

5

Lorie Theisen

Injuries to blood vessels rarely occur independent of injuries to other structures of the hand (i.e., bone, tendon, nerve, and blood vessels). However, it is worthwhile to singularly examine the operative and postoperative management of repaired blood vessels. Keep in mind these other repaired structures and incorporate the appropriate postoperative management guidelines. It is important for the treating therapist to receive information from the surgeon regarding tension and patency of the anastomosed vessel as well as the integrity of other repaired structures. The postoperative course must then be modified for the individual case.[1]

Generally the greatest amount of healing, in the vascular system, occurs within the first 4 weeks postoperatively.[2] More specifically, healing of the endothelial lining, a single cell layer of the vessel wall serving as a permeable barrier between the blood and other cells of the vessel, occurs in the first 2 weeks. Simultaneously, proliferation of the intimal smooth muscle cells occurs, adding structural integrity. Remobilization is initiated after endothelial healing has occurred and therefore should not interfere with or cause excessive intimal thickening.[3]

DEFINITION

Surgical procedure for restoration of blood supply.

SURGICAL PURPOSE

Vessel repair is a common procedure used to restore circulation to a part deprived of its blood supply (Fig. 5-1). This includes both veins and arteries. Often magnification or the operating microscope is used to per-

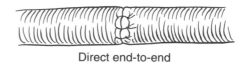

Direct end-to-end

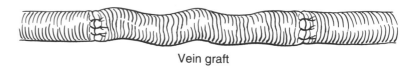

Vein graft

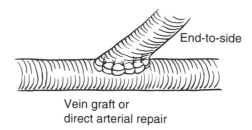

End-to-side

Vein graft or
direct arterial repair

Fig. 5-1. Vessel repair restores circulation to a part deprived of its blood supply.

form these repairs. If direct artery to artery or vein to vein repair cannot be accomplished, vein grafts are used to bridge the gap. Frequently other adjacent structures such as nerve, bone, muscle, or skin may be damaged. Treatment of these injuries will also be required.

TREATMENT GOALS

Maintain integrity of vessel repair while addressing other specific problems of the injured hand, such as joint stiffness or tendon/soft tissue tightness.

POSTOPERATIVE INDICATIONS/PRECAUTIONS FOR THERAPY

I. Indications
   Rehabilitation may be indicated following the surgical repair of the vessel for protective splinting, remobilization, and education.
II. Precautions
   A. Follow precautions identified from the surgeon regarding specifics of the vessel repair.

B. Avoid extremes in temperature to avoid triggering vascular spasm. Arterial spasm can lead to ischemia.[4]
C. Avoid excessive external compression or pressure via dressing, splints, etc.
D. Therapy is not indicated where thrombosis or the integrity of the vessel is in question.
E. Avoid trauma to the soft tissues, especially when removing any dressing.
F. Vigorous exercise that causes pain may precipitate vasospasm.
G. Exercise or splints should not decrease digital temperatures. It is recommended that these temperatures be monitored closely.[5]

POSTOPERATIVE THERAPY

I. Elevation of the injured part above the heart, but the elbow should not be flexed more than 30 degrees. Excessive elevation should be avoided if there is arterial congestion.[6]
II. Application of protective splinting to preserve the arches of the hand and to preserve maximum ligament length of any immobilized joint, with consideration given to other injuries such as tendon laceration, nerve laceration, fractures, etc.
III. Observe carefully for signs of vascular compromise, which may include an increase in edema, a decrease in temperature, an increase in pain, and a dusky appearance.
IV. Therapy is initiated between 2 to 4 weeks following surgical repair. Treatment should address problems identified at the initial evaluation such as joint tightness, soft tissue tightness, adhesions preventing tendon gliding, sensory dysfunction, edema, etc.
V. Continue to instruct the patient in restrictions identified by the surgeon, such as no smoking or caffeine.

POSTOPERATIVE COMPLICATIONS

I. Arterial occlusion
II. Venous congestion
III. Severe edema
IV. Infection
V. Cold intolerance

EVALUATION TIMELINE

I. Initial evaluation at 2 to 4 weeks postoperatively should include assessment of range of motion (ROM), edema, sensibility, and temperature.
II. Progress evaluation every 2 weeks thereafter.
III. Gross grasp and prehension strength evaluation may be performed at

10 weeks postoperatively, providing guidelines/precautions of other repaired structures are met.

REFERENCES

1. Goldner R: Post-operative management. p. 205. In Urbaniak J (ed): Hand Clinics Microvascular Surgery. Vol. 1. No. 2. WB Saunders, Philadelphia, 1985
2. Kader P: Therapists management of the replanted hand. p. 821. In Hunter J (ed): Rehabilitation of the Hand: Surgery and Therapy. 3rd Ed. CV Mosby, St. Louis, 1990
3. Wilgis EFS: Ischemic conditions of the upper extremity. p. 4991. In McCarthy J (ed): Plastic Surgery: The Hand. Vol. 8. WB Saunders, Philadelphia, 1990
4. Chase R: Microsurgery. p. 360. In: Atlas of Hand Surgery. Vol. 2. WB Saunders, Philadelphia, 1984
5. Steichen J, Idler R: Surgical aspect of replantation and revascularization. p. 801. In Hunter J (ed): Rehabilitation of the Hand: Surgery and Therapy. 3rd Ed. CV Mosby, St. Louis, 1990
6. Koman LA: Diagnostic study of vascular lesions. p. 219. In Urbaniak J (ed): Hand Clinics. Vol. 1. No. 2. WB Saunders, Philadelphia, 1985

SUGGESTED READING

Brand P: External stress: effect at the surface. p. 88. In: Clinical Mechanics of the Hand. CV Mosby, St. Louis, 1985

Nerve Repair

6

Beth Farrell

Peripheral nerves activate the intricately balanced muscles in the upper extremity that enable hand function. With nerve loss, this balance is lost and permanent hand deformities can occur. Therapy following nerve repair is critical for restoring hand function. Goals of therapy are to maintain joint range of motion (ROM), prevent permanent deformities, promote normal sensibility, and restore upper extremity strength and function.

Nerve repairs are initially seen in therapy 1 to 2 weeks following surgery for fabrication of a protective splint. Active ROM (AROM) and passive ROM (PROM) of the interphalangeal (IP) joints is initiated at about 2 weeks. Care is taken to protect a nerve repair by maintaining joint extension for radial nerve repairs and wrist flexion and metacarpal joint flexion for median and ulnar nerve repairs.[1,2] Wrist ROM is initiated at 4 weeks following surgery. Dynamic splinting, for joint tightness, may be used at 7 weeks postoperatively. Strengthening can begin between 9 and 12 weeks, and sensory re-education should be initiated as soon as moving and constant touch are perceived at the fingertips of the involved digit(s).[3] Refer to the sensory re-education guideline for a detailed program for regaining sensibility. It should be noted, however, that all patients suffering from peripheral nerve loss should be instructed on compensatory techniques for protecting the desensate extremity from extreme temperatures and other painful stimuli.

The following protocol presents as a guideline for treating patients suffering from peripheral nerve interruption. The addendum section describes the effects of nerve lesions on motor function.

DEFINITION

Approximation of the ends of a lacerated nerve (Fig. 6-1)

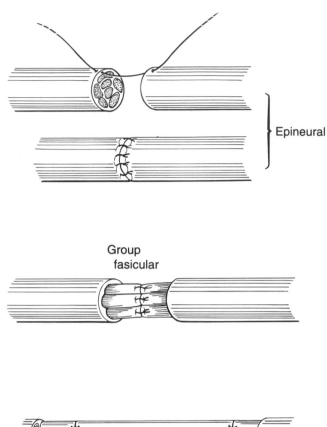

Epineural

Group
fasicular

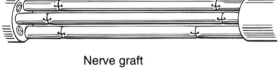

Fig. 6-1. Approximated ends of a
lacerated nerve.

Nerve graft

TREATMENT AND SURGICAL PURPOSE

To protect against damage and deformity within the defined territory of
the injured nerve prior to its maximum recovery. The goal of surgery is to
restore nerve continuity by direct repair or nerve grafting in order that an
optimum number of nerve fibers will reach their appropriate sensory and/
or motor end organs. During the preoperative and postoperative periods,
appropriate monitoring and therapy is required to optimize the final result.
Patience on the part of those treating or being treated is necessary because
of the slow rate of nerve healing.

TREATMENT GOALS

I. Restore motor function.
II. Restore sensibility.
III. Minimize recovery time.
IV. Maximize functional recovery. Expected rate of recovery time for nerve repairs is 1 in per month.[4]
V. Maintain ROM of all upper extremity joints during nerve recovery period.
VI. Provide appropriate preoperative care for delayed repairs or grafts. See section on Postoperative Care with Flexor Tendon Involvement.

POSTOPERATIVE INDICATIONS AND PRECAUTIONS

I. Indications
   A. Primary nerve repair: indicated for a clean, sharply cut nerve in which the damaged ends can be seen and approximated. This type of nerve repair is performed immediately following an injury or within 1 to 3 weeks.[1]
   B. Secondary nerve repair: usually indicated in the presence of a severely crushed or avulsed nerve. This surgery involves recutting the nerve and removal of the neuroma 3 to 6 weeks following injury.[1]
   C. Nerve grafts: usually performed when a direct repair cannot be done without tension or nerve condition is poor. It is often done as a secondary procedure.
II. Precautions
   A. Fractures/dislocations
   B. Stretching of the nerve beyond its elastic limit
   C. Loss of sensation, which could cause secondary injury

POSTOPERATIVE THERAPY FOR PRIMARY OR SECONDARY REPAIR

I. Ulnar and median nerve repairs at the wrist level
   A. 0 to 6 days: rest in dressing with wrist flexed at 30 degrees.
   B. 7 days: position hand in dorsal protection splint with wrist flexed at 30 degrees (Fig. 6-2). For lacerations within the proximal half of the forearm the elbow is splinted in flexion also. Include a C-bar on the protection splint for median nerve injuries to prevent thumb adduction contracture, active IP motion.
   C. 2 weeks: remove sutures. Begin active and passive flexion and extension of IP joints with wrist in flexed position. Begin scar management if wound is healed.

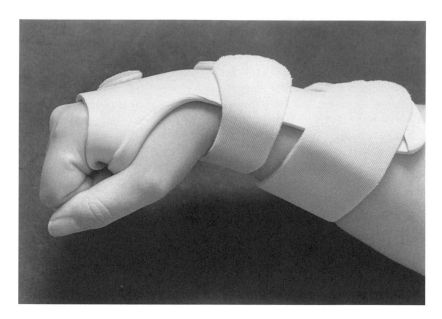

Fig. 6-2. Splinting for wrist level lacerations of median or ulnar nerve.

D. 3 weeks: position wrist in neutral. The test to determine rate of extension splinting is to check for complaints of burning and tingling when gently extending the wrist. Once elicited, shape the splint prior to that point of extension.

E. 4 weeks: begin ROM of wrist. Avoid symptoms of irritability. For more proximal lesions in which the elbow was immobilized, begin ROM of elbow when the symptoms are not elicited upon mobilization.

F. 5 weeks: splint only at night and in crowds. Children need to be protected for about 1 week longer than adults. For ulnar nerve lesions, position the hand in a lumbrical block splint to wear during the day and evening.[1] For median nerve repair, if needed, the patient should wear a separate C-bar splint when not wearing a protective splint.[1]

G. 6 weeks: begin wrist extension with fingers extended. Evaluate sensibility. Begin sensory re-education and desensitization program when appropriate. (Refer to sensory evaluation guideline, Ch. 7.)

H. 7 weeks: dynamic splint, if necessary, for joint tightness.

I. 9 to 12 weeks: begin strengthening/work rehabilitation.

II. Radial nerve repair for forearm and above

A. 0 to 6 days: rest in dressing with wrist extended.

B. 7 to 14 days: position hand in forearm based static wrist extension splint with dynamic extension outriggers for fingers and thumb.[1] If lesion more proximal, the elbow should be immobilized.

C. 2 weeks: remove sutures. Begin active and passive flexion and extension of IP joints with metacarpophalangeal (MCP) joints and wrist in extension. Begin friction massage on scar and encourage

patient to perform this several times daily, gradually increasing intensity as tolerated. Apply a gel sheet or an elastomer mold to scar once wound is healed.
  D. 4 weeks: begin ROM of wrist with fingers extended.
  E. 7 weeks: dynamic splint, if necessary, for joint tightness.
  F. 9 to 12 weeks: begin strengthening/occupational training.

PREOPERATIVE CARE FOR DELAYED PRIMARY REPAIR OR NERVE GRAFT

I. Goals of therapy
  A. Full PROM: provide patient with home exercise program to be performed several times a day.
  B. Minimal tendon adherence in the scar: achieved through active movement and scar management techniques.
  C. Promote good skin condition: massage with cream several times daily.
  D. Patient education to avoid injury from sharp objects, heat, pressure areas.
    1. Teach patient to compensate visually for loss of protective sensation.
    2. Have patient wear warm gloves in winter.
    3. Use long-handled cooking utensils.

POSTOPERATIVE CARE WITH FLEXOR TENDON INVOLVEMENT

This is essentially the same as for nerve repair without tendon involvement, except that active flexion of the fingers is postponed until the third or fourth week. Active flexion is performed with the MCP joints in flexion. The major postoperative complication in nerve repair with tendon involvement is flexor tightness of the wrist due to tendon adherence. To help overcome this, scar management techniques are emphasized. Also, finger flexion exercises should be stabilized and performed individually.

POSTOPERATIVE THERAPY FOR NERVE GRAFTS

I. Treatment
  A. 0 to 9 days: wrist is held in neutral, elbow in slight flexion.
  B. 10 days: dressing removed, sutures removed, if needed. Begin very gentle AROM and PROM.[1,5]
  C. 4 weeks: should expect an advancing Tinel's sign. Begin more progressive AROM and PROM.
  D. 5 weeks: treated like a nerve repair. Refer to the appropriate nerve repair treatment sections.

POSTOPERATIVE COMPLICATIONS

I. Severe edema
II. Infection
III. Neuromas
IV. Secondary deformity
V. Severe pain (if noted during ROM exercises, may indicate over-stretching of the nerve)
VI. Intraneural fibrosis
VII. Hand burns and/or cuts due to loss of protective sensation

EVALUATION TIME LINE

Evaluations	Time Line
Wound condition	7 days
Edema	7 days
Range of motion	10–14 days
Sensory	6–8 weeks
Manual muscle test	3 months

For sensory and manual muscle testing, re-evaluate once every 6 to 8 weeks thereafter.

ADDENDUM

I. Effects of nerve lesion on motor function[6,7]
    A. High radial nerve lesion
        1. Wrist drop due to paralysis of wrist extensors.
        2. Diminished abduction and extension of thumb due to paralysis of abductor pollicis longus (APL) and extensor pollicis brevis (EPB).
        3. Inability to extend MCP joints due to paralysis of the long extensors.
        4. Weak grasp and pinch due to the inefficiency of the unopposed long flexors (shortened).
        5. Loss of sensation of the lateral two-thirds of the dorsum of the hand and a portion of the thenar eminence area, as well as the dorsum of the proximal phalanges of the lateral three and one-half fingers.
        6. Weakened supination due to paralysis of the supinator muscle.
    B. Posterior interosseus nerve: presents with the same effects as above, except that sensation is not lost and wrist extension is present, but weakened.

C. Ulnar nerve lesion at the wrist.
1. Loss of adduction and abduction of the fingers due to paralysis of interossei.
2. Hyperextension of fourth and fifth MCP joints with flexion of the IP joints due to unopposed action of the extensor digitorum communis (EDC).
3. Weak thumb adduction due to paralysis of adductor pollicis (AdP).
4. Loss of opposition of the fifth finger due to paralysis of the opponens digiti quinti.
5. Weak thumb opposition due to paralysis of the AdP.
6. Weak MCP flexion due to paralysis of the third and fourth lumbricales.
7. Weak pinch due to paralysis of the AdP, deep head of the flexor pollicis brevis (FPB), and the first dorsal interosseous.
8. Weak grasp due to paralysis of the interossei, third and fourth lumbricales, and the flexor digitorum profundus (FDP) of the fourth and fifth fingers.
9. Sensory nerve loss of volar and dorsal aspects of the medial third of the hand, little finger, and ulnar half of the ring finger.

D. Ulnar nerve lesion in the proximal forearm presents with these additional problems.
1. Weak IP flexion of IP joints of fourth and fifth fingers due to paralysis of the ulnar half of the FDP.
2. Weak wrist flexion due to paralysis of the flexor carpi ulnaris (FCU).

E. Median nerve lesion in the proximal forearm
1. Weak forearm pronation due to paralysis of pronator teres
2. Weak wrist flexion due to paralysis of flexor carpi radialis (FCR)
3. Weak finger flexion due to paralysis of flexor digitorum superficialis (FDS)

F. Anterior interosseous nerve (proximal one-third of forearm)
1. Loss of distal interphalangeal (DIP) joint flexion of the index and middle fingers due to paralysis of FDP to each of these digits
2. Loss of thumb IP joint flexion due to paralysis of flexor pollicis longus (FPL)
3. Weak forearm pronation due to paralysis of pronator quadratus

G. Palmar branch of the median nerve (wrist level)
1. Sensory loss of the central palm area and the palmar surfaces of the lateral three and one-half digits
2. Weak MCP joint flexion of index and middle fingers due to paralysis of the first two lumbricals
3. Weak pinch due to paralysis of opponens pollicis (OP), abductor pollicis brevis (APB), and the superficial head of the FPB
4. Loss of thumb palmar abduction due to paralysis of the APB

REFERENCES

1. Wilgis EF: Nerve repair and grafting. p. 915. In Green DP (ed): Operative Hand Surgery. 2nd Ed. Vol. 2. Churchill Livingstone, New York, 1988
2. Trombly CA: Occupational Therapy for Physical Dysfunction. 2nd Ed. p. 357. Williams & Wilkins, Baltimore, 1983
3. MacKinnon SE, Dellon AL: Surgery of the Peripheral Nerve. Thieme Medical Publishers, Inc., New York, 1988
4. Hopkins HL, Smith HD: Willard and Spackman's Occupational Therapy. 6th Ed. p. 468. JB Lippincott, Philadelphia, 1983
5. Omer GE, Spinner M: Management of Peripheral Nerve Problems. WB Saunders, Philadelphia, 1980
6. Lampe EW: Clinical Symposium: Surgical Anatomy of the Hand. p. 10. New Jersey Pharmaceutical Division, CIBA-GEIGY Corporation, 1988
7. Tam AM: Nerves. p. 12-1. In Kasch MC, Taylor-Mullins PA, Fullenwider L (eds): Hand Therapy Review Course Study Guide. Hand Therapy Certification Commission, Garner, NC, 1990

SUGGESTED READINGS

Arsham NZ: Nerve injury. p. IV. In Ziegler EM (ed): Current Concepts in Orthotics: A Diagnosis-Related Approach to Splinting. Rolyan Medical Products, Chicago, 1984
Boscheinen MJ, Davey V et al: The Hand: Fundamentals of Therapy. p. 60. Butterworth Publishers, Cambridge, 1985
Sunderland S: Nerves and Nerve Injuries. 2nd Ed. Churchill Livingstone, New York, 1978

Sensory Evaluation 7

Mallory S. Anthony

The ability of the hand to function, and to interact and explore the environment is dependent upon good sensibility. The complexity of the sensory system makes the comprehensive sensory evaluation a challenge to the clinician, and creates the need for a battery of tests to provide more accurately a true sensory picture.

The peripheral nerve is composed of motor, sensory, and sympathetic nerve fibers. The sensory evaluation is aimed at examining the sympathetic and sensory nerve fiber integrity. The cell body of the presynaptic sympathetic nerve fibers lies in the anterior horn of the spinal cord, and the postsynaptic sympathetic nerve fibers originate in the neurons of the ganglion located from T_1 to T_7. These unmyelinated fibers will innervate the skin, blood vessels, and hair follicles. The cell body of the sensory nerve fibers lies in the dorsal root ganglia. These sensory nerve fibers terminate in the skin as free nerve endings or end in a number of specialized receptors.

Nerve fibers are either myelinated or unmyelinated and vary in diameter size. Fibers of smaller diameter regenerate ahead of larger fibers. In the case of nerve compression, the larger myelinated fibers are most sensitive to ischemia and are affected first.

Much controversy exists concerning the neurophysiologic basis of sensory testing. Dellon has done considerable research in this area and outlines end-organ specific tests based on type of stimulus and slowly or rapidly adapting properties of receptors. For example, static two-point is used to test Merkle cell-neurite complex (slowly adapting) and moving two-point is used to test rapidly adapting Pacinian and Meissner corpuscles. Others believe that many of these end organs may respond to both high and low frequency stimuli, thereby making specific end-organ testing difficult.[1] Also, to further compound this issue, the lack of control of certain variables in our testing compromises accuracy. For example, the difficulty in controlling the velocity and application of force in two-point discrimination and vibration testing (tuning forks) make the results less reliable. Further investigation is needed to help clarify these controversial issues and further study is needed to improve the reliability of our testing instruments.

Our goals and selection of evaluation tools vary, depending on whether we are examining a nerve compression lesion or a nerve repair.

In mild nerve compression, symptoms may only be elicited with provocative tests. Since nerve compression causes changes in threshold (i.e., the stimulus intensity required to elicit the normal response is altered), a hypersensitive response may also be present in mild compression. Later in the course of nerve compression the threshold appears to be raised, so that a greater stimulus intensity is required to elicit the same response as before the injury.[2] Threshold tests such as vibration and Semmes–Weinstein monofilaments (touch/pressure) are used to assess this sensory change.

With further compression, and loss of nerve fibers due to Wallerian degeneration, the sensory system will have a diminished number of nerve fibers innervating an area. This decrease in innervation density can be measured by two-point discrimination testing, both moving and static.[2]

In patients following nerve repair, our goals and sensory assessment are directed toward monitoring axonal regeneration and reinnervation into distal tissue. This will help us evaluate sensory function and indicate the need to begin re-education when necessary.

Factors that affect recovery following nerve repair are (1) time interval between injury and repair, (2) state of stumps at suture line, (3) postoperative stretching and suture line tension, and (4) patient's potential for healing (age, metabolic and nutritional status).[3] The normal rate of axonal regeneration is 1 to 5 mm/day or 1 in/month if conditions are optimal.

The following protocol is designed to present the components of a comprehensive sensibility evaluation and offer guidelines for the selection of appropriate tests.

DEFINITION

I. Sensation: the conscious perception of basic sensory input. This is what we re-educate.[4]
II. Sensibility: neural events occurring at the periphery, nerve fibers, nerve receptors. This is what we evaluate.[4]
    A. Protective sensibility: return of sensibility as evidenced by the ability to perceive pinprick, touch, and temperature.
    B. Functional sensibility: return of sensibility to a level that enables the hand to engage in full activities of daily living, including those in which vision is occluded while the hand manipulates an object.[5]
    C. Hierarchy of sensibility capacity.[6]
        1. Detection: most simple level of function. Requires that the patient be able to distinguish a single point stimulus from nor-

mally occurring atmospheric background stimulation (threshold tests).

2. Discrimination: the ability to perceive that stimulus A differs from stimulus B. Involves the capacity to detect each stimulus as a separate entity and to distinguish between them (two-point discrimination tests).

3. Quantification: involves organizing tactile stimuli according to degree. For example: the patient selects which texture is roughest, most irregular, or smooth. (Some sensory re-education techniques incorporate this concept.)

4. Recognition: most complicated level of function. The ability to identify objects, vision occluded. (Some sensory re-education techniques incorporate this concept as well as the Dellon modification of Moberg pick-up test.)

III. Tactile gnosis: object identification as related to the peripheral nervous system.

IV. Stereognosis: refers to central nervous system (CNS) recognition of objects (cortical).

V. Sensory evaluation: the testing of hand sensibility.

TREATMENT PURPOSE

Nerve injuries or conditions that involve the sensory fibers going to the hand will leave a region of altered sensibility. This sensory deficit may fit a specific pattern. In some cases it is important to document such deficiencies. Documentation of these sensory losses may be important in determining an accurate diagnosis or monitoring the progression of healing in an impaired nerve.

TREATMENT GOALS

I. Determine the presence of changes in sensibility for nerve compression.

II. Determine if axonal regeneration is occurring following nerve repair.

III. Determine the sequence of recovery of sensory submodalities as a guide to instituting sensory re-education, following nerve repair.

IV. Determine the status of sensibility in a way that reflects hand function.

INDICATIONS/PRECAUTIONS FOR EVALUATION

I. Indications
   A. Peripheral nerve repair, digital nerve repair
   B. Nerve compressions: contusions
   C. Replants
   D. Resurfaced flaps, grafts, and cross-finger flaps

    E. Brachial plexus injuries

    F. Crush injuries

II. Precautions

    A. Underlying vascular or neuropathic disease, which could lead to nerve ischemia and dysfunction

    B. Fatigue

    C. Negative attitude and decreased motivation

    D. Pain/hypersensitivity

    E. Excessive callous formation on area being tested

    F. A distracting or cold testing environment

THERAPY (EVALUATION)

I. Patient history

    A. Name, age, sex, dominance, occupation

    B. Date, nature, and level of injury

    C. Subjective report of symptoms and what aggravates or relieves these symptoms

    D. Brief assessment of motor function (include grip and pinch), because motor function may affect performance on certain sensibility tests

    E. Patient's medical status

II. Examination of sympathetic function

    A. Vasomotor changes

        1. Temperature, color, and edema (initial warm phase: cold intolerance)

    B. Sudomotor changes

        1. Lack of sweating in autonomous area of sympathetic fibers after denervation

        2. May have increased sweating with nerve irritation

    C. Pilomotor changes

        1. Absence of gooseflesh response with complete interruption of sympathetic supply

    D. Trophic changes

        1. Skin texture: thin and smooth.

        2. Atrophy of finger pulps with long-term denervation.

        3. Nail changes: striations, ridges, increased hardness.

        4. Hair growth: may fall out in region of denervation or may become longer, finer. May demonstrate increased hair growth (hypertrichosis).[5]

        5. Increased susceptibility to injury with slowed healing due to atrophy of epidermis and decreased nutrition and vascularity.[5]

III. Classification of sensibility tests

    A. Objective tests: require only passive cooperation of the patient, not his subjective interpretation of a stimulus.[5]

        1. Ninhydrin test

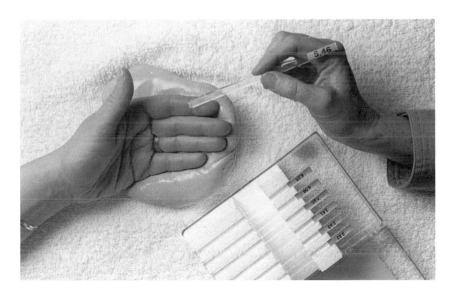

Fig. 7-1. Semmes–Weinstein monofilaments.

    2. O'Riain wrinkle test
    3. Electrodiagnostic tests
B. Threshold tests: determine minimum stimulus that can be perceived by patient.
    1. Pain and temperature (heat/cold)
    2. Touch/pressure (Semmes–Weinstein monofilaments) (Fig. 7-1)
    3. Vibration (Fig. 7-2)

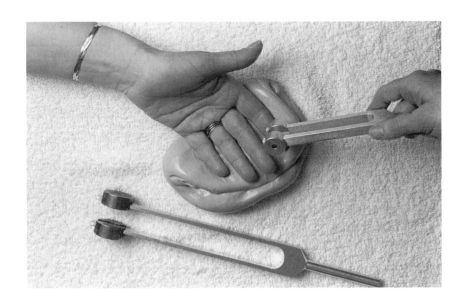

Fig. 7-2. Tuning forks may be used for vibratory testing.

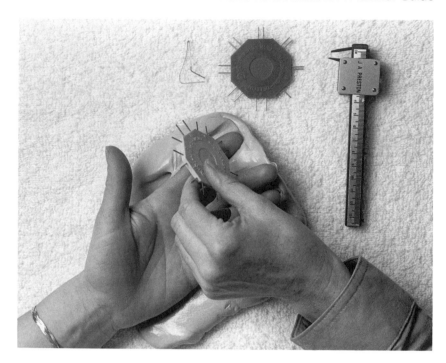

Fig. 7-3. Devices that may be used to assess two-point discrimination.

C. Functional tests: assess the quality of sensibility.
    1. Moving two-point discrimination (Fig. 7-3)
    2. Static two-point discrimination
    3. Localization
    4. Dellon modification of Moberg pick-up test
    5. Moberg pick-up test
IV. Testing variables
  A. Testing environment: *quiet,* free from distraction.
  B. Patient: *relaxed* and able to concentrate.
  C. Be aware of differences between *testing instruments.*
  D. Use *standardized method* of testing.
  E. *Same examiner* should perform successive tests on a given patient.
  F. Patient's hand should be *fully supported* in examiner's hand or in putty (or similar medium).
V. Testing techniques
  A. Standard tests
    1. Tinel's sign
      a. Present at site of nerve compression lesion.
      b. Used to monitor level of regenerating sensory axons.
      c. Difficult to test if too much muscle lies over the nerve.
    2. Provocative tests
      a. Direct pressure over suspected compression site.
      b. Manipulation of the extremity to render the nerve locally ischemic, for example, wrist flexion (Phalen's test) (Fig.

7-4) for median nerve compression at wrist [carpal tunnel syndrome (CTS)], elbow flexion for ulnar nerve compression at elbow (cubital tunnel) (Fig. 7-5), forearm pronation with wrist flexion and ulnar deviation for radial sensory nerve compression[2] (Fig. 7-6).

3. Pain assessment
   a. Intensity (rating scale from "no pain" to "unbearable pain")
   b. Location (map out or describe painful area)
   c. Frequency
   d. Type (burning, throbbing, aching, stabbing, tingling, cramping, etc.)
   e. Factors that increase or decrease pain
   f. Other factors (e.g., patient taking pain medication)

4. Semmes-Weinstein monofilaments
   a. Used as a stimulus to establish the threshold of touch ranging from light touch (a necessary component of fine discrimination) to deep pressure (a form of protective sensation).
   b. Helpful in monitoring return of sensibility in the early months after nerve repair and helpful in assessing early changes in sensibility caused by nerve compression.
   c. The technique and procedure for administering the Semmes–Weinstein monofilaments test is described in detail in Reference 7.

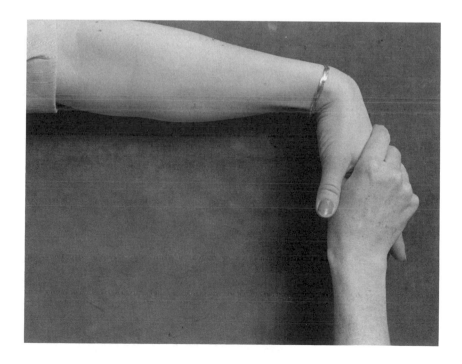

Fig. 7-4. Phalen's test.

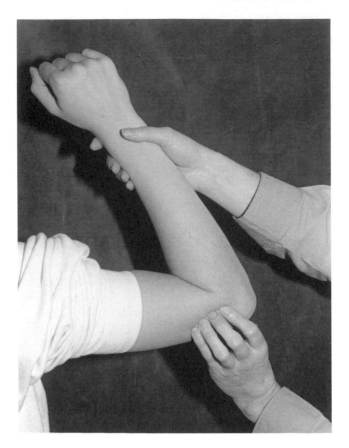

Fig. 7-5. Provocative test for ulnar nerve at elbow (cubital tunnel).

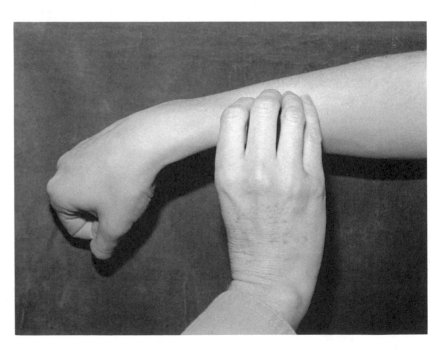

Fig. 7-6. Provocative test for radial sensory nerve compression.

      d. Interpretation of test results, as well as a systematic work sheet to document findings and color code results, can be found in appendix 7-1 and 7-2.

5. Vibration 30 cps.

      a. Useful in diagnosing digital nerve injuries, in which a perceived difference in vibration exists between the two tested autonomous zones of the digit.

      b. Useful in detecting earliest sensory changes in nerve compression, since the large group A beta fibers, which carry the perceptions of light touch and vibration, are affected first by the ischemia.

         i. The fingertips of the thumb and index are test sites in median nerve compression.

         ii. The tip of the small finger is the test site for ulnar nerve compression.

      c. It is useful following nerve repair to document return of vibration to the affected area. When 30 cps reaches palm, may begin early phase sensory re-education.

      d. Patient should localize the stimulus because perception of the stimuli may occur through an adjacent peripheral field of a noninjured nerve, for example, radial nerve with a median nerve injury.[3]

      e. The technique and procedure for administering vibration testing is described in Reference 3. The pronged end of the tuning fork is applied to the test site, as suggested by Dellon, because the fingertips have a significant amount of subcutaneous tissue and a more intense stimulus is needed, especially when the threshold level is raised. Also, tuning fork should be warmed prior to testing, as patient may react to the coldness rather than vibration.

6. Vibration: 256 cps.

    Same as described under 30 cps

7. Moving touch (as described by Dellon)

      a. Used to test return of light and heavy movement following nerve repair.

      b. Helps to determine when to begin early phase sensory re-education.[3]

      c. Technique (unpublished protocol and Reference 8). Both light and heavy movement are tested using middle finger to stroke small areas of the extremity, above and below nerve repair site, moving proximal to distal along dysfunctioning nerve distribution. Light versus heavy refers to intensity of the stimulus.

      d. Procedure (unpublished protocol and Reference 8). The patient is instructed to close his eyes and then respond to the moving stimulus by indicating whether or not the stimulus was felt and if so, where. Responses for both light and heavy movement are documented on the sensory evaluation form with appropriate symbols, and a description of "feeling" is recorded.

8. Constant touch (as described by Dellon)
   a. Used to test return of light and heavy touch following nerve repair.
   b. Helps to determine when to begin late phase sensory re-education.
   c. Technique (unpublished protocol and Reference 8). Both light and heavy touch are tested using middle finger to touch different areas on the extremity above and below the nerve repair site, moving proximal to distal along dysfunctioning nerve distribution. Each stimulus should be maintained for no longer than one-half second. Light versus heavy refers to the intensity of the pressure applied.
   d. Procedure; Same as described under moving touch.

9. Moving two-point discrimination
   a. A measure of innervation density (number of functioning nerve fiber-receptors for a given area), and a measure of hand function requiring moving touch,[9,10] for example, object identification (tactile gnosis) and fine manipulative tasks (such as buttoning a button).
   b. Tested when moving touch is perceived at the fingertip, following nerve repair.[3]
   c. Normal values are elevated in later stages of nerve compression (due to decrease in innervation density).
   d. According to methods described by Dellon[3,10]:
      i. Testing is begun with instrument set between 6 and 8 mm distance between the two points.
      ii. The instrument is moved proximally to distally on the fingertip parallel to the long axis of the finger with the testing ends side by side.
      iii. The pressure used is just light enough so that the patient can perceive the stimulus without discomfort (skin blanching itself is not a guide to stimulus intensity).
      iv. The patient is required to respond accurately to two out of three stimuli before the distance is narrowed.[10]
   e. The same two-point device should be used for all testing as the terminal probes can produce significant variations in response.[11,12] Ends should be blunt to ensure testing of touch not pain.
   f. Moving two-point discrimination returns earlier than static two-point (following nerve repair), approaching normal 2 to 6 months before static two-point.[3]
   g. Values for normal and abnormal moving two-point discrimination can be found in appendix 7-3 (key section of sensory evaluation form).

10. Static two-point discrimination.
  a. A measure of innervation density; assesses patient's ability to perform tasks requiring precision grip[10] (i.e., holding a pencil to write or a needle to sew).
  b. Tested when constant touch is perceived at the fingertip, following nerve repair.[3]
  c. Normal values are elevated in later stages or nerve compression (due to decrease in innervation density).
  d. According to methods described by Dellon[3,10]:
    i. Testing is begun with instrument set between 6 and 8 mm distance between the two points.
    ii. The instrument is placed on the fingertip parallel to the long axis of the finger (testing ends lie proximal/distal).
    iii. The pressure used is the same as for moving two-point discrimination.
    iv. The patient is required to respond accurately to two out of three stimuli before the distance is narrowed.[10]
  e. The same two-point device should be used for all testing, as the terminal probes can produce significant variations in response.[11,12] Ends should be blunt to ensure testing of touch not pain.
  f. Static two-point discrimination recovers 2 to 6 months slower than moving two-point, and is therefore a later assessment of discrimination.
  g. Values for normal and abnormal static two-point discrimination can be found in appendix 7-3 (key section of sensory evaluation form).
11. Localization of touch
  a. A more integrated level of perception than simple recognition of stimulus.
  b. May be tested while assessing recovery of vibration, touch/pressure, and two-point discrimination.
  c. May be tested and recorded as a separate function, that is, recording both the site of stimulation and the patient's perceived site of referral on a drawing of the hand (e.g., a touch stimulus to the index may be perceived in the thumb tip).
  d. The patient's record of localization is useful in planning a sensory re-education program.

B. Additional functional and objective tests
  1. Moberg pick-up test
    The patient is asked to pick up a number of everyday objects and put them into a small box, first with involved hand, then with uninvolved, both with eyes open, then eyes closed. Time required and manner of prehension are noted.[3,5,13]

    2. Dellon modification of Moberg pick-up test
       a. Dellon has modified Moberg's test by standardizing the items used and requiring identification of them.
       b. Objects of similar material are used to avoid giving clues by texture or temperature, and objects are graded to require increasing ability to discriminate.
       c. Specific testing technique and procedure can be found in references 3 and 5.
    3. Ninhydrin test
       a. An objective test of sympathetic function most helpful when testing children, patients with language problems, or malingerers.
       b. The test identifies areas of decreased sweat secretion after peripheral nerve disruption: the Ninhydrin Spray turns purple when it reacts with amino acids in sweat.
       c. Specific technique and procedure can be found in References 13 and 14.
       d. Frequently parallels recovery of pain and temperature (i.e., protective sensation).[3]
       e. Does not correlate with return of sensory function.
    4. O'Riain wrinkle test
       a. An objective test that identifies areas of denervation (i.e., denervated skin does not wrinkle, as does normal skin when soaked in warm water).
       b. Specific technique and procedure can be found in References 14 and 15.
       c. Does not correlate with return of sensory function.
VI. Recommendations for test selection.
  A. Compression syndromes
    1. Provocative tests: Tinel's
    2. Nerve conduction testing to detect early sensory changes
    3. Vibration tests
    4. Semmes–Weinstein to detect early changes in touch-pressure perception (threshold changes)
    5. Static and moving two-point discrimination to detect advanced sensory changes
  B. Nerve repair
    1. Examination of hand for sympathetic dysfunction.
    2. Tinel's to determine level of regenerating axons.
    3. Vibration (30 cps), moving touch, constant touch, and vibration (256 cps).
    4. Semmes–Weinstein monofilaments to help assess quality of touch return.
    5. When return of touch reaches fingertips, static and moving two-point on fingertips, with localization of touch over entire area of dysfunction, will determine level of functional return.
    6. Moberg pick-up or Dellon modification.

POSTOPERATIVE COMPLICATIONS

I. Neuroma
II. Continued decrease in sensibility
III. Continued hypersensitivity (see protocol on desensitization)

EVALUATION TIMELINE

I. Nerve repair
   A. Baseline evaluation at 6 to 8 weeks post-operatively.
   B. Re-evaluation every 6 to 8 weeks.
   C. Begin desensitization and re-education when appropriate (as described in the following protocols).

REFERENCES

1. Bell-Krotoski JA: Sensibility testing: state of the art. p. 575. In Hunter JM, Schneider LH, Mackin EJ, Callahan AD (eds): Rehabilitation of the Hand: Surgery and Therapy. 3rd Ed. CV Mosby, St Louis, 1990
2. MacKinnon SE, Dellon AL: Classification of nerve injuries as the basis for treatment. p. 35. In: Surgery of the Peripheral Nerve. 1st Ed. Thieme Medical Publishers, New York, 1988
3. Dellon AL: Evaluation of Sensibility and Re-education of Sensation in the Hand. Williams & Wilkins, Baltimore, 1981
4. MacKinnon SE, Dellon AL: Sensory rehabilitation after nerve injury. p. 521. In: Surgery of the Peripheral Nerve. 1st Ed. Thieme Medical Publishers, New York, 1988
5. Callahan AD: Sensibility testing: clinical methods. p. 594. In Hunter JM, Schneider LH, Mackin EJ, Callahan AD (eds): Rehabilitation of the Hand: Surgery and Therapy. 3rd Ed. CV Mosby, St. Louis, 1990
6. Fess EE: Documentation: essential elements of an upper extremity assessment battery. p. 53. In Hunter JM, Schneider LH, Mackin EJ, Callahan AD (eds): Rehabilitation of the Hand: Surgery and Therapy. 3rd Ed. CV Mosby, St. Louis, 1990
7. Bell-Krotoski JA: Light touch-deep pressure testing using Semmes-Weinstein monofilaments. p. 585. In Hunter JM, Schneider LH, Mackin EJ, Callahan AD (eds): Rehabilitation of the Hand: Surgery and Therapy. 3rd Ed. CV Mosby, St. Louis, 1990
8. Dellon AL, Edgerton MT: Evaluating recovery of sensation in the hand following nerve injury. Hopkins Med J 130:235, 1972
9. MacKinnon SE, Dellon AL: Diagnosis of nerve injury. p. 65. In: Surgery of the Peripheral Nerve. 1st Ed. Thieme Medical Publishers, New York, 1988
10. Dellon AL, MacKinnon SE, Crosby PM: Reliability of two-point discrimination measurements. J Hand Surg 12A:693, 1987
11. Crosby PM, Dellon AL: Comparison of two-point discrimination testing devices. Microsurgery 10:134, 1989
12. Levin LS, Regan N, Pearsall LG, Nunley JA: Variations in two-point discrimination as a function of terminal probes. Microsurgery 10:236, 1989

13. Moberg E: Objective methods for determining the functional value of sensibility in the hand. J Bone Joint Surg 40B:454, 1958

14. Phelps PE, Walker E: Comparison of the finger wrinkling test results to establish sensory tests in peripheral nerve injury. Am J Occup Ther 31:565, 1977

15. O'Riain S: New and simple test of nerve function in the hand. Br Med J 3:615, 1973

SUGGESTED READINGS

Dellon AL: Sensory recovery in replanted digits and transplanted toes: a review. J Reconstr Microsurg 2:123, 1986

Dellon AL: "Think Nerve" in upper extremity reconstruction. Clin Plast Surg 16: 617, 1989

Dellon AL: Sensibility testing. p. 135. In Gelberman RH (ed): Operative Nerve Repair and Reconstruction. JB Lippincott, Philadelphia, 1991

Eversmann WW: Compression and entrapment neuropathies of the upper extremity. J Hand Surg 8:759, 1983

Louis DS, Greene TC, Jacobson KE et al: Evaluation of normal values for stationary and moving two-point discrimination in the hand. J Hand Surg 9A:552, 1984

MacKinnon SE, Dellon AL: Two-point discrimination tester. J Hand Surg 10A: 906, 1985

Melzack R, Wall PD: On the nature of cutaneous sensory mechanisms. Brain 85: 331, 1962

Omer GE: Nerve response to injury and repair. p. 515. In Hunter JM, Schneider LH, Mackin EJ, Callahan AD (eds): Rehabilitation of the Hand: Surgery and Therapy. 3rd Ed. CV Mosby, St. Louis, 1990

Szabo RM, Gelberman RH, Dimick MP: Sensibility testing in patients with carpal tunnel syndrome. J Bone Joint Surg 66A:60, 1984

Tubiana R: Examination of the Hand and Upper Limb. WB Saunders, Philadelphia, 1984

Waylett-Rendall J: Sequence of sensory recovery: a retrospective study. J Hand Ther 2:245, 1989

Werner JL, Omer GE: Evaluating cutaneous pressure sensation of the hand. Am J Occup Ther 24:347, 1970

Appendix 7-1

INTERPRETATION OF TEST RESULTS—SEMMES–WEINSTEIN

Normal touch: is a recognition of light touch, and therefore deep pressure is also within normal limits. This level is the most significant of all levels because it allows the examiner to distinguish between areas of normal and areas of sensory diminution.

Diminished light touch: if a patient has diminished light touch, provided his motor status and cognitive abilities are in play, has fair use of his hand, his graphesthesia and stereognosis are both close to normal and adaptable, has good temperature appreciation, has good protective sensation, and most often two-point discrimination is fair to good, he may not realize that he has had a sensory loss.

Diminished protective sensation: if a patient has diminished protective sensation, he will have diminished use of his hand, difficulty in manipulating some objects, a tendency to drop some objects, and he may complain of weakness of his hand; but, he will have an appreciation of pain and temperature and this should help him from injuring himself, and he may have some manipulative skills.

Sensory re-education can begin at this level.

Loss of protective sensation: if a patient has loss of protective sensation, he will have a diminished, if not absent, temperature appreciation. He will have a tendency to injure himself easily and it may even be dangerous for him to be around machinery. He will be able to feel a pin prick and have deep pressure sensation, which does not make him totally asensory. Instructions on protective care are helpful to prevent injury.

Untestable: he may or may not feel a pin prick, but will have no other discrimination of levels of feeling. If a patient feels a pin prick in an area otherwise unstable, it is important to note this during the mapping. Instructions on protective care of the hand are mandatory at this level to prevent the normally occurring problems associated with the asensory hand.

Further interpretation of the effect the decrease or loss of sensibility has on patient function depends on the area and the extent of loss whether musculature is diminished.

(From Bell-Krotoski,[7] with permission.)

Appendix 7-2

UPPER EXTREMITY ASSESSMENT BATTERY

SENSORY EVALUATION:
SEMMES-WEINSTEIN CALIBRATED MONOFILAMENTS

PALMAR/DORSAL (circle):

DATE:	THUMB 1 U - R	INDEX 2 U - R	LONG 3 U - R	RING 4 U - R	SMALL 5 U - R
1					
2					
3					
4					
5					
6/7	////	6 _		6 _	

PALMAR/DORSAL (circle):

DATE:	THUMB 1 U - R	INDEX 2 U - R	LONG 3 U - R	RING 4 U - R	SMALL 5 U - R
1					
2					
3					
4					
5					
6/7	////	6 _		6 _	

PALMAR/DORSAL (circle):

DATE:	THUMB 1 U - R	INDEX 2 U - R	LONG 3 U - R	RING 4 U - R	SMALL 5 U - R
1					
2					
3					
4					
5					
6/7	////	6 _		6 _	

KEY:*

		Filament	Pressure (gm/mm²)
	Normal	1.65-2.83	1.45- 4.86
Blue	Diminished light touch	3.22-3.61	11.1 - 17.7
Purple	Diminished protective sensation	3.84-4.31	19.3 - 33.1
Red	Loss of protective sensation	4.56-6.65	47.3 -439.0
Red-lined	Untestable	6.65	439.0

*Levine, S., Pearsall, G., & Ruderman, R.: J Hand Surg, 3:211, 1978.

NAME_____

NUMBER_____

HAND_____

(From Fess,[6] with permission.)

Appendix 7-3

THE UNION MEMORIAL HOSPITAL BALTIMORE, MARYLAND 21218	DATE	IMPRINT WITH PATIENT CHARGE PLATE
HAND SENSIBILITY EVALUATION		

Diagnosis: _____ Date & Type of Operation _____

_____

SUBJECTIVE COMPLAINTS

_____

_____

RIGHT   LEFT

TWO-POINT DISCRIMINATION

	R MOVING	STATIC (WEBER)	L MOVING	STATIC (WEBER)
THUMB				
INDEX				
3RD				
4TH				
5TH				

COMMENTS:

KEY

xx	30 c.p.s.	
" "	256 c.p.s.	
—	Light Movement	
= =	Heavy Movement	
°°	Light Touch	
®®	Heavy Touch	
X	Tinel's	

Two-Point (Static)
2-6 mm	Normal
7-10 mm	Fair
11-15 mm	Poor
16 mm	Non-Functional

Two-Point (Moving)
2-3 mm	Normal
4-6 mm	Fair
7-9 mm	Poor

Semmes-Weinstein
1.65-2.83 mg	Normal
3.22-3.61 mg	Diminished Light Touch
3.84-4.31 mg	Diminished Protective
4.56-6.65 mg	Loss of Protective
6.65 mg	Untestable

Therapist's Signature

License No.

Appendix 7-4

SENSORY TESTING (A GENERAL GUIDELINE)

Sensory Level	Tests	Test Results	Additional Tests	Functional Level
Untestable	Pin Prick or Semmes-Weinstein 6.65	Negative Response	—	Nonfunctional Protective Care Instruction Mandatory
Loss of protective	Pin Prick or Semmes-Weinstein 4.56–6.56	Positive Response	Vibration Temperature	Tendency to Injure Hand Protective Care Instruction Helpful
Decreased protective	Semmes-Weinstein (SW)	Possible Hypersensitivity 3.84–4.31 SW	—	Decreased Use of Hand Some Manipulative Skills Tendency to Drop Objects
Diminished light touch	Semmes-Weinstein (SW)	3.22–3.61 SW	Moberg Pick-Up Test or Dellon Modification	Fair Use of Hand Close to Normal Graphesthesia and Tactile Gnosis
Moving touch out to fingertips	Moving Two-Point Discrimination	7–9 mm (poor) 4–6 mm (fair)	Moberg Pick-Up Test or Dellon Modification	Fair Use of Hand Good Hand Function and Tactile Gnosis May Still Drop Objects
Constant touch out to fingertips	Static Two-Point Discrimination	11–15 mm (poor) 7–10 mm (fair)	Moberg Pick-Up Test or Dellon Modification	Fair Use of Hand Good Hand Function
Normal sensation	Moving Two-Point Static Two-Point Semmes-Weinstein	2–3 mm 2–6 mm 2.36–2.83	— — —	Return to Normal Level of Function

Desensitization

8

Mallory S. Anthony

Hypersensitivity often occurs after hand trauma. The patient experiences an exaggerated, painful response to a normally nonpainful stimuli, at or near the injury site. (This hypersensitivity should not be confused with the general manifestations of pain, as seen in causalgia or the shoulder–hand syndrome.) Desensitization techniques are used to diminish symptoms of hypersensitivity and are designed to gradually increase the patient's tolerance for touch to the area. Desensitization techniques are identical in concept to sensory re-education. Instead of the patient learning to associate an old name with a new pattern of transmitted impulses to identify an object he is touching, the patient is learning to filter out the unpleasant sensations to permit perception of the underlying meaningful sensory input.[1] This is re-education of unpleasant sensations instead of re-education of touch.

The following protocol suggests several techniques, based on the use of graded stimuli, beginning with nonirritating media and progressing to stronger types of stimulation.

DEFINITION

I. Hypersensitivity: a condition of extreme discomfort or irritability in response to normally nonnoxious tactile stimulation.
II. Desensitization: the use of modalities and procedures designed to reduce the symptoms of hypersensitivity.

TREATMENT PURPOSE

To gradually increase the patient's tolerance to tactile stimulation in an area of hypersensitivity.

TREATMENT GOALS

To help patient achieve maximal level of function by increasing his tolerance to touch in the hypersensitive area.

INDICATIONS/PRECAUTIONS FOR THERAPY

I. Indications
   A. Neuromas
   B. Sensitive amputated tips (stumps)
   C. Hypersensitive scars and surrounding areas
   D. Nerve injuries with dysesthesia (a painful and persistent sensation induced by a gentle touch of the skin)
II. Precautions
   A. Diffuse pain
   B. Areas with open wounds
   C. Deep pain not remediated with desensitization

THERAPY

I. Desensitization program
   A. Treatment time: 5 to 10 minutes (stop when stimulus becomes noxious), three to four times per day.
   B. Demonstrate technique on self or patient's noninvolved side.
   C. May need to protect the area initially (splint with bubble, gel sheet, elastomer, cuff of lambswool).

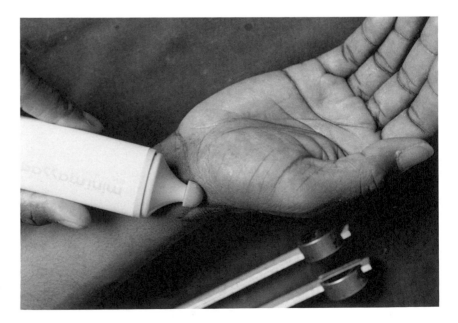

Fig. 8-1. Graded vibration can range from tuning fork to battery or electric powered vibrators.

D. The less irritating stimulus should feel comfortable before advancing to a more irritating stimulus.
II. Techniques (based on a hierarchy of least irritating stimulus to most)
A. Vibration
1. Graded uses of vibration can range from tuning fork to battery or electric powered vibrators with various shaped attachments and varying speeds (Fig. 8-1).
2. Progression can range from stimulating only the periphery of the hypersensitive area, to intermittent stimulation of actual area, to continuous contact with actual area as tolerance allows.
B. Texture
1. Graded textures can be used to stroke and tap the hypersensitive area.
2. The following list is a suggested guideline of progression:
a. Cotton
b. Lambswool
c. Felt
d. Orthopaedic felt (⅛ in)
e. Orthopaedic felt (¼ in)
f. Terrycloth towel
g. Velcro loops
h. Velcro hook or fine grades of sandpaper (Fig. 8-2)
C. Immersion particles
1. Immersion of the involved hand into a number of containers filled with particles ranging from least irritating to most

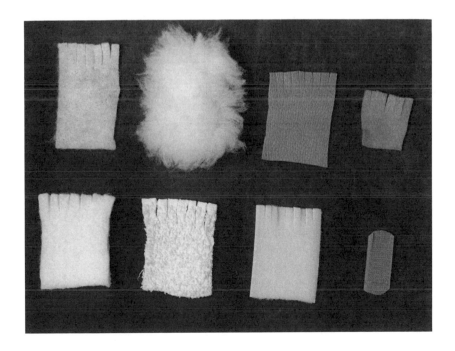

Fig. 8-2. Examples of graded textures to be used in hypersensitive areas.

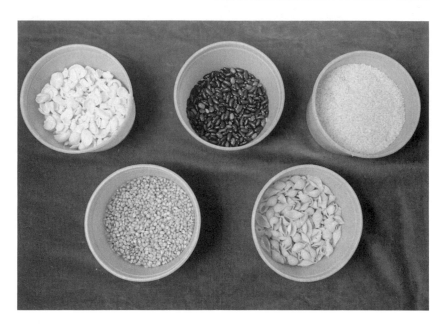

Fig. 8-3. Examples of particle media.

2. The following is a suggested list of particle media (Fig. 8-3)
   a. Cotton
   b. Styrofoam pieces
   c. Sand
   d. Beans
   e. Popcorn
   f. Rice
   g. Macaroni
D. Maintained pressure
   1. The use of continuous mild pressure with an isotoner glove, or gelsheet, or elastomer mold can also increase comfort in hypersensitive area.
   2. Progress treatment using varying degrees of pressure over area, including weight-bearing pressure as patient tolerates.
E. Other modalities to decrease hypersensitivity
   1. Massage
   2. Tapping
   3. Transcutaneous electrical nerve stimulator (TENS) directly on or adjacent to hypersensitive area (Fig. 8-4).
   4. Fluidotherapy (Fig. 8-5)
   5. Moist heat for relaxation
F. Therapeutic activities to regain confidence and restore function
   1. Theraplast and exercises for strengthening.
   2. Work simulation and/or craft activities (Fig. 8-6).
   3. Resume re-education if necessary, after hypersensitivity is gone.

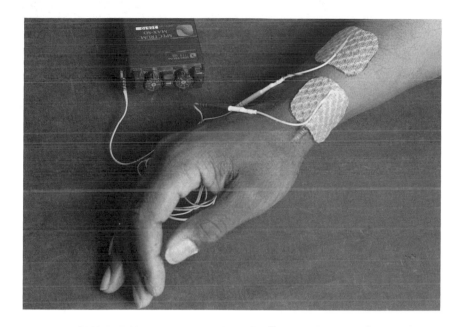

Fig. 8-4. TENS used to decrease hypersensitivity.

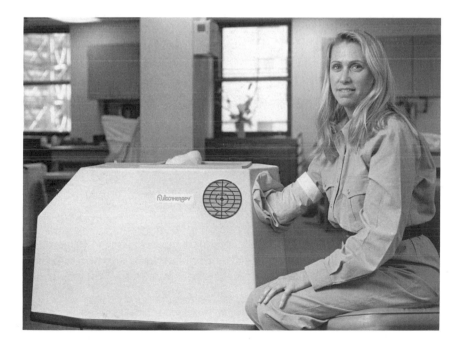

Fig. 8-5. Fluidotherapy.

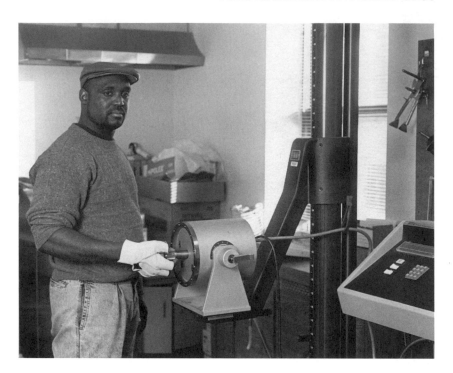

Fig. 8-6. Work simulation to regain confidence and restore function.

COMPLICATIONS THAT MAY CAUSE HYPERSENSITIVITY

1. Nerve regeneration without an intact endoneural tube
II. Scar formation of regenerating axons with or without constriction
III. Neuroma formation
IV. Adherence of nerve to its bed
V. Constriction of blood flow causing ischemic pain

EVALUATION TIMELINE

Initially, patient should be rechecked two to three times per week for treatment, assessment, and home program reviews. Gradually decrease frequency of visits as patient feels comfortable with home program and shows improvement. Then recheck once per month until discharge.

REFERENCE

1. MacKinnon SE, Dellon AL: Sensory rehabilitation after nerve injury. p. 521. In: Surgery of the Peripheral Nerve. 1st Ed. Thieme Medical Publishers, New York, 1988

SUGGESTED READINGS

(Please also refer to Sensory Evaluation Suggested Readings)

Barber LM: Desensitization of the traumatized hand. p. 721. In Hunter JM, Schneider LH, Mackin EJ, Callahan AD (eds): Rehabilitation of the Hand: Surgery and Therapy. 3rd Ed. CV Mosby, St. Louis, 1990

Hardy MA, Moran CA, Merritt WH: Desensitization of the traumatized hand. Virginia Med 109:134, 1982

Melzack R: The puzzle of pain. Basic Books, New York, 1973

Wilson RL: Management of pain following peripheral nerve injuries. Orthop Clin North Am 12:343, 1981

Wolpe J: Systematic desensitization. J Nerve Ment Dis 132:189, 1961

Sensory Re-education 9

Mallory S. Anthony

Following peripheral nerve repair, the transmission of neural impulses is altered (due to factors discussed under postoperative complications) for sensory perception in the somatosensory cortex. When a patient attempts to interpret, at a conscious level, this altered profile of neural impulses, he must match the current profile to his memory of profiles stored in some "association" cortex. If no match is made, the altered profile of sensory impulses may be ignored, or the patient may not know what he has felt. Sensory re-education is an attempt to give the patient a new set of matching profiles.[1,2]

Re-education requires a patient who is intelligent, motivated, and willing to make a conscious effort to incorporate the involved hand into daily activities and to carry out a structured program on a daily basis. In this way, through the use of higher cortical functions (attention, learning, memory), a patient can learn to compensate for sensory deficits.[3]

The following treatment protocol is a guideline. There is no one technique for sensory re-education. The timing for the exercises is determined by the pattern of sensory recovery.

DEFINITION

Sensory re-education is a method by which the patient learns to interpret the pattern of abnormal sensory impulses generated after an interruption in the peripheral nervous system.

TREATMENT PURPOSE

Following injury to sensory nerves the pattern of recovery is variable and never returns to normal. Only some sensory fibers reach their proper end organs and therefore the territory of reinnervation is incomplete. In order to help the patient with rehabilitation, he is trained to recognize the altered sensory feedback to the brain and interpret the sensory stimulus.

TREATMENT GOALS

I. To teach the patient who lacks protective sensation guidelines for protecting the hand against stress during everyday function activities.
II. To guide patient in early and late re-education to maximize hand function, and help patient achieve the fullest functional potential provided by nerve repair.

INDICATIONS/PRECAUTIONS FOR THERAPY

I. Indications
   A. Patient in whom protective sensation is lacking or severely decreased as evidenced by inability to perceive potentially harmful stimuli (pinprick, deep pressure, hot/cold, repetitive low-grade friction).[3]
   B. Patients who have protective sensation but lack discriminative sensation (i.e., localization, two-point discrimination, and tactile gnosis).[3]
II. Precautions
   Sensory re-education cannot be applied to a painful, hypersensitive, stiff, or swollen upper extremity.[2]

POSTOPERATIVE THERAPY

I. Home program
   A. Patient should practice re-education exercises 5 minutes, three to four times per day.
   B. Patient should not stimulate the involved hand directly with the uninvolved hand as he will receive two sets of sensory information, one from each hand, and this will be confusing.[1]
   C. Any interested individual (spouse, other family members, friends) can be shown sensory re-education exercises to help the patient with home program.

II. Patients who lack protective sensation should be instructed in the following guidelines, suggested by Anne Callahan,[3] to help them compensate.[4]
   A. Avoid exposure of involved area to heat, cold, and sharp objects.
   B. Be conscious of not applying more force than necessary when gripping a tool or object.
   C. Note that the smaller the handle, the less distribution of pressure over the gripping surfaces. Avoid using small handles by building them up whenever possible.
   D. Avoid tasks that require use of one tool for long periods of time, especially if the hand is unable to adapt by changing the manner of grip.
   E. Change tools frequently at work to rest tissue areas subject to pressure.
   F. Observe the skin for signs of stress (i.e., redness, swelling, warmth) from excessive force or repetitive pressure. Rest the hand if these signs occur.
   G. If blisters, lacerations, or other wounds occur, treat them with the utmost care to avoid further injury to the skin and possible infection.
   H. Keep skin soft. Follow a daily routine of skin care including soaking and oil (or lotion) massage to hold in moisture.
III. Early phase re-education: begin when 30 cps vibration and/or moving touch have returned to an area, for example, the palm.[1]
   A. To re-educate specific perceptions (i.e., movement versus constant touch, sharp versus dull).
   B. To re-educate incorrect localization (where is stimulus perceived in reference to site of stimulation).
   C. Suggested techniques[1-4]
      1. Use fingertip or pencil eraser (blunt surface) (Fig. 9-1).
      2. Press hard enough for patient to feel stimulus.
      3. Perform moving and/or constant touch to palm or finger when these submodalities reach the area.
      4. The patient observes what is happening (moving versus constant, sharp versus dull, location of stimulus), shuts his eyes and concentrates on what he is perceiving, then opens his eyes to confirm what is happening.
      5. If patient incorrectly identifies the stimulus, repeat process.
   D. Evaluate progress with accuracy of response, mapping of localization, Semmes–Weinstein monofilaments, and/or vibration testing (preferably vibrometer).
IV. Late phase re-education: begin when moving and constant touch, and/or 256 cps vibration can be perceived at the fingertips with good localization.
   A. To guide patient in recovery of tactile gnosis.
   B. Suggested techniques.[1-4]
      1. Exercises should be graded beginning with the discrimination of larger objects, with greater differences among them in size,

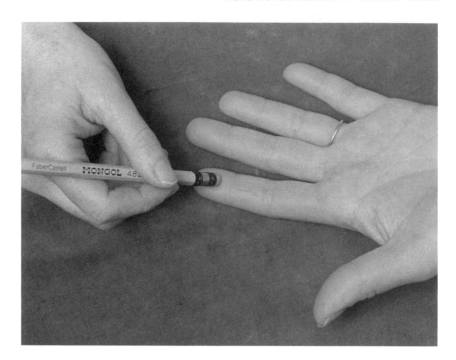

Fig. 9-1. Blunt surface used for sensory re-education in early phase.

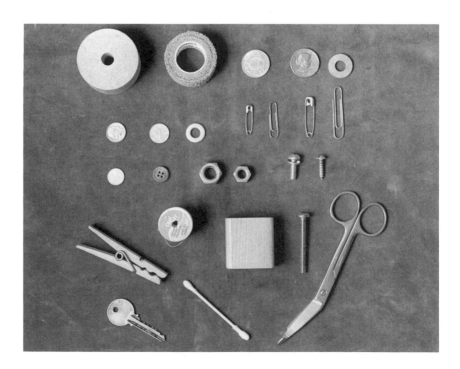

Fig. 9-2. Graded object discrimination to recover tactile gnosis.

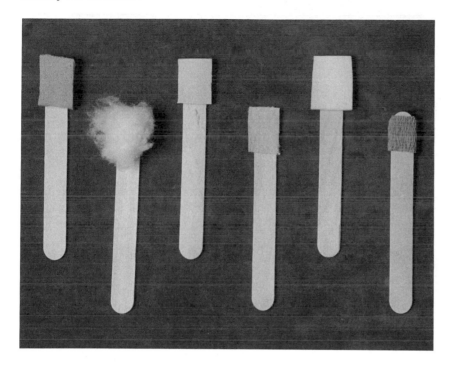

Fig. 9-3. Textures may be used for late phase re-education.

shape, and texture, progressing to more subtle differences (Fig. 9-2).

2. Discrimination of various textures (Fig. 9-3), as well as object identification using a set of familiar household objects, can be used for re-education.

3. The sequence of object (or texture) grasp with eyes open, then shut with concentration of perception, then eyes open for reinforcement, is used.

C. Accuracy of response (i.e., number of correctly identified objects or textures) is recorded. Time to perform the task may also be recorded.

D. Moving and static two-point discrimination should be tested periodically to assess sensory status.

V. Other techniques of re-education.

A. Graphesthesia: therapist traces a number, letter, or geometric figure on involved area and patient tries to identify it.[3]

B. Bilateral exercises can be used by having the patient differentiate between various textures of material or sandpaper with vision, then vision occluded.[7]

C. Patients can be asked to pick out and identify an object in a bowl of sand, rice, or beans with vision occluded (Fig. 9-4)

D. Activities that duplicate or incorporate work activities should be included in patient's therapy to practice specific sensory grips and prepare patient for previous work.

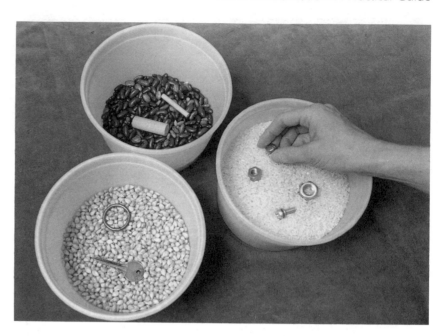

Fig. 9-4. Locating and identifying objects imbedded in various media.

POSTOPERATIVE COMPLICATIONS THAT MAY REQUIRE RE-EDUCATION

I. Axons may regenerate to an irreversibly degenerated end organ.
II. Axons may arrive at correct digital area, but reinnervate the wrong end organ.
III. Axons may never re-enter distal endoneurial sheath.
IV. Axons may be misdirected to the wrong finger.

EVALUATION TIMELINE

Initially, patient should be checked in the clinic once per week for several weeks, for sensory assessment and home program review. As patient feels comfortable with home program, decrease the frequency of treatment. Check patient every 6 to 8 weeks for sensory evaluation and any necessary changes in re-education program.

REFERENCES

1. Dellon AL: Evaluation of Sensibility and Re-education of Sensation in the Hand. Williams & Wilkins, Baltimore, 1981
2. MacKinnon SE, Dellon AL: Sensory rehabilitation after nerve injury. p. 521. In: Surgery of the Peripheral Nerve. 1st Ed. Thieme Medical Publishers, New York, 1988

3. Callahan AD: Methods of compensation and reeducation for sensory dysfunction. p. 611. In Hunter JM, Schneider LH, Mackin EJ, Callahan AD (eds): Rehabilitation of the Hand: Surgery and Therapy. 3rd Ed. CV Mosby, St Louis, 1990

4. MacKinnon SE, Dellon AL: Appendix E: Sensory re-education protocols. p. 589. In: Surgery of the Peripheral Nerve. 1st Ed. Thieme Medical Publishers, New York, 1988

SUGGESTED READINGS

(Please also refer to Sensory Evaluation Suggested Readings)

Dellon AL, Jabaley MF: Reeducation of sensation in the hand following nerve suture. Clin Orthop 163:75, 1982

Omer GE: Sensation and sensibility in the upper extremity. Clin Orthop Relat Res 104:30, 1974

Extensor Tendon Repair 10

Barbara Rabinowitz

Both static and dynamic therapeutic approaches to extensor tendon injuries are described. For the uncomplicated extensor tendon injuries in zones V, VI, and VII the static approach is most often utilized. If the surgeon requests the metacarpophalangeal (MCP) joint to be splinted statically at 20 degrees to 30 degrees of flexion to retain the integrity of the collateral ligaments,[1] it may be appropriate to use the dynamic method to prevent extensor lag. The dynamic method may also facilitate a better outcome in the complicated extensor tendon injury, which is defined as including injury to the periosteum of bone, extensor retinaculum, or adjacent soft tissues.[1]

When progressing a patient using either method, it is important to have a "feel" of the tendon. When there is a developing MCP extensor lag, this would indicate a longer course of MCP extension splinting to be balanced with MCP flexion as permitted by tendon healing. Conversely, if the problem is decreased MCP flexion and/or extrinsic extensor tendon tightness, dynamic MCP flexion splinting may be indicated when the extensor tendon is strong enough to tolerate this.

What follows are two methods of extensor tendon rehabilitation. It is important to keep abreast of further research in tendon healing and postoperative treatment to facilitate the best outcome for each patient.

DEFINITION

Primary repair of complete rupture or laceration of any digital extensor tendon in zones V, VI, or VII and thumb extensors zones T–III, T–IV, T–V.

SURGICAL PURPOSE

To restore continuity and maintain gliding of the extensor mechanism from the metacarpal phalangeal joints proximally toward the wrist level. These tendons, which are at least nine in number, excluding the wrist extensors, travel through six separate compartments over the distal radius before they fan out over the dorsum of the hand, toward each individual digit (Fig. 10-1). Tendon gliding is critical beneath the retinacular liga-

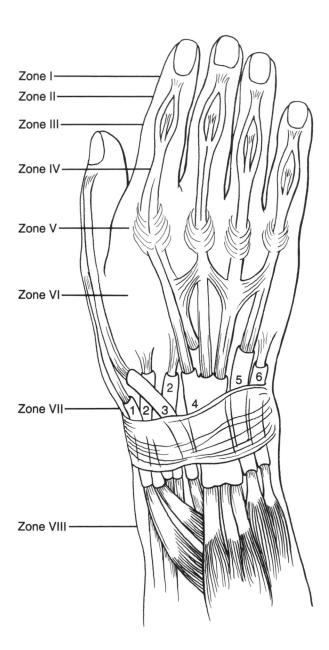

Fig. 10-1. Dorsal compartments through which extensors travel.

ments covering these fibrosseous compartments at the wrist. Scarring over the dorsal surface of the hand is a problem because of scant soft tissue protection between the skin's surface and the underlying skeletal structures. Tendon suturing techniques may vary depending on the zone where the actual juncture is placed. The zone of tendon division may not coincide with the actual skin laceration. Other than lacerations, extensor tendon continuity may be lost secondary to attrition from sharp bone fragments after fracture, rheumatoid arthritis, tendinitis, and developmental absence.

TREATMENT GOALS

    I. Prevent tendon rupture and extensor lag
   II. Promote tendon healing
  III. Encourage tendon gliding
  IV. Restore active range of motion (AROM) and passive range of motion (PROM)
   V. Edema control
  VI. Pain control
 VII. Scar management
VIII. Maintain full range of motion (ROM) of all uninvolved joints of the affected upper extremity
  IX. Return to previous level of function

POSTOPERATIVE INDICATIONS/PRECAUTIONS FOR THERAPY

  I. Indications
     Surgical repair of finger extensor tendons in zones V, VI, VII, and/or thumb extensors in zones T–III, T–IV, or T–V
 II. Precautions
   A. Infection
   B. Combined flexor tendon repair
   C. Fractures
   D. Extreme pain
   E. Severe edema

POSTOPERATIVE THERAPY

  I. Static method
   A. Finger extensors: zones V, VI, and VII
     1. Immediately postoperatively
       Static volar extension splint wrist 30 degrees to 45 degrees extension, MCP joints 0 degrees to 30 degrees flexion accord-

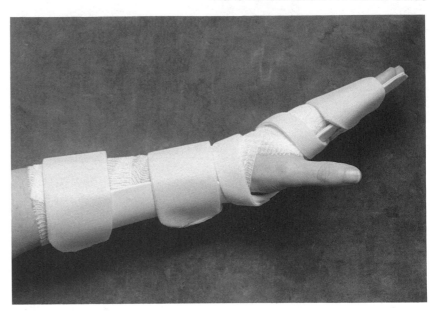

Fig. 10-2. Static postoperative protection splint for fingers.

ing to physician's preference, interphalangeal (IP) joints full extension (Fig. 10-2).
2. 2 weeks
   a. Shorten splint at distal interphalangeal (DIP) level (if MCP joints splinted at 0 degrees).
   b. Keeping wrist and MCP joints in full passive extension, allow active isolated DIP flexion and extension with therapist supervision.
3. 3 weeks
   a. Shorten splint to allow proximal interphalangeal (PIP) motion.
4. 4 weeks
   a. Remove splint several times a day to allow active MCP flexion and extension with wrist passively maintained in extension.
   b. Keep wrist and MCP joints splinted between exercise sessions.
5. 5 weeks
   a. Shorten splint to allow MCP motion.
   b. Remove splint several times a day to allow active protected wrist motion.
6. 6 weeks
   a. Decrease wrist splint use.
7. 7 weeks
   a. Passive isolated flexion of wrist, MCP, and IP joints may be initiated.

8. 8 to 10 weeks
    a. Regain full active flexion and extension.
    b. Gentle resistive exercises may be initiated.
9. 10 to 12 weeks
    a. Full activity may be resumed.
B. Thumb zones T–III, T–IV, and T–V
  1. *Immediately postoperatively*
    a. Static volar splint with wrist 30 degrees to 40 degrees of dorsiflexion, carpometacarpal (CMC) in extension with slight abduction (dependent upon tension on tendon repair). Check with surgeon. MCP and IP in extension (Fig. 10-3).
  2. 3 weeks
    a. Shorten splint to allow flexion of the IP joint.
    b. Active extension exercises of the IP joint are begun. Other joints remain immobilized to protect the tendon repair.
  3. 4 weeks
    a. Static splinting is decreased.

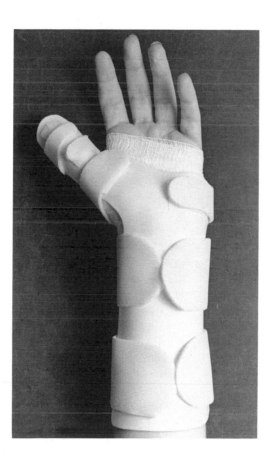

Fig. 10-3. Static postoperative protection splint for thumb.

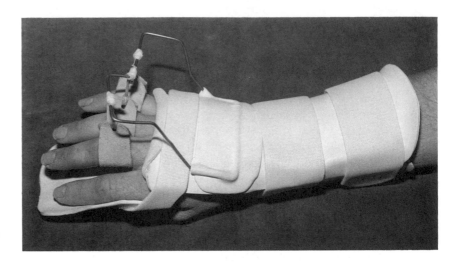

Fig. 10-4. Splint for dynamic treatment of finger extensor repairs in zones V, VI, and VII.

      b. Active flexion and extension exercises of the MCP and IP joints are emphasized.

      c. If an active extension lag is noted, dynamic splinting should be considered for use periodically during the day.

   4. 5 weeks

      a. Active full excursion flexion is initiated.

      b. Isolated passive joint flexion is initiated.

   5. 7 to 8 weeks

      Gentle resistive exercises may begin.

II. Dynamic method: The following guidelines have been described by Evans.[1]

   A. Finger extensors: zones V, VI, VII.

     1. 3 days postoperatively

      a. Splint with dorsal forearm based dynamic extension component with wrist at 40 degrees to 45 degrees extension, MCP and IP joints rest at 0 degrees dynamic traction and an interlocking forearm based palmar blocking component that permits approximately the following degrees of active flexion at the MCP joints (Fig. 10-4).

        i. index: 28 degrees

        ii. middle: 27 degrees

        iii. ring: 41 degrees

        iv. small: 38 degrees

      b. Exercise

        i. Active flexion to limits of volar splint, and passive extension via dynamic extension component. Repeat 10 times each waking hour.

      c. Digital static extension splints may be used in conjunction with above splint in order to maintain PIP and DIP joints at 0 degrees and facilitate active motion at the MCP level.

2. Patient followed in therapy for
   a. Wound care.
   b. Splint adjustments.
   c. Controlled passive motion to the IP joints while maintaining wrist and MCP joints in extension. Allow 45 degrees of IP motion for zone V and 60 degrees of IP motion for zone VI.
3. 3 to 6 weeks
   a. Splint
      i. Day: volar block removed and continue with dorsal dynamic splint.
      ii. Night: wear volar and dorsal splint components.
   b. Exercise
      Begin gradual active motion of MCP and IP joints.
4. 6 to 12 weeks
   Same as static method
B. Thumb extensors, zones T–IV and T–V
   1. 3 days postoperatively
      a. Dorsal forearm based splint with wrist extended 30 degrees to 45 degrees, CMC joint in neutral, MCP and IP joints 0 degrees via dynamic extension traction combined with a forearm based palmar blocking splint allowing 60 degrees active MCP flexion (Fig. 10-5).
      b. Exercise
         Active MCP joint flexion to limits of volar splint and passive extension via dynamic extension component
   2. 3 to 12 weeks.
      Same as dynamic finger extensor guidelines.

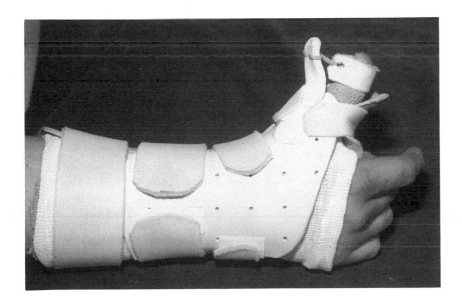

Fig. 10-5. Splint for dynamic treatment of thumb extensor repair in zones T–IV and T–V.

POSTOPERATIVE COMPLICATIONS

I. Tendon rupture
II. Excessive scar formation
III. Active extensor tendon lag
IV. Extrinsic extensor tendon tightness limiting composite flexion

EVALUATION TIMELINE

I. 4 weeks: AROM MCP and IP joints
II. 5 weeks: AROM wrist
III. 7 weeks: PROM and AROM wrist, MCP and IP joints
IV. 10 weeks: Strength; re-evaluate ROM and strength measurements every 4 weeks

REFERENCE

1. Evans RB: Therapeutic management of extensor tendon injuries. p. 492. In Hunter JM, Schneider LH, Mackin EJ, Callahan AD (eds): Rehabilitation of the Hand. 3rd Ed. CV Mosby, St. Louis, 1990

SUGGESTED READINGS

Dovelle S, Heeter PK: Early controlled mobilization following extensor tendon repair in zone V-VI of the hand: Preliminary report. Contemp Orthop II(4):41, 1985

Dovelle S, Heeter PK, Fischer DR, Chow JA: Rehabilitation of extensor tendon injury of the hand by means of early controlled motion. Am J Occupat Ther 43(2):115, 1989

Evans RB: Management of the healing tendon . . . What must we question? J Hand Ther 2:61, 1989

Evans RB, Burkhalter WE: A study of the dynamic anatomy of extensor tendons and implications for treatment. J Hand Surg 11A(5):774, 1986

Hunter JM, Schneider LH, Mackin EJ (eds): Tendon Surgery in the Hand. CV Mosby, St. Louis, 1987

Kuxhaus M: Flexor and extensor tendon repairs. p. 49. In Ziegler EM (ed): Current Concepts in Orthotics: A Diagnosis-Related Approach to Splinting. Roylan Medical Products, Menomonee Falls, 1984

Rosenblum NI, Robinson SJ: Advances in flexor and extensor tendon management. p. 17. In Muran CA (ed): Hand Rehabilitation. Churchill Livingstone, New York, 1986

Rosenthal EA: The extensor tendons. p. 458. In Hunter JM, Schneider LH, Mackin EJ, Callahan AD (eds): Rehabilitation of the Hand. 3rd Ed. CV Mosby, St. Louis, 1990

Flexor Tendon Repair   **11**

Barbara Rabinowitz

The following is a treatment approach that combines early controlled passive motion[1] and early controlled mobilization with elastic traction and active extension.[2] It focuses primarily on zone II injuries of the digits and addresses the primary goals of preventing tendon rupture, encouraging tendon gliding, and preventing flexion contractures.

Digital zones III, IV, V may be treated the same or three and one-half weeks of immobilization may be used initially.[3]

Treatment for flexor pollicus longus repairs is essentially the same as digital tendon lacerations except that the position of the rubber band (if used) should be directed toward the ulnar side of the wrist.[4]

DEFINITION

Primary and delayed primary repair of complete rupture or laceration of digital flexor tendons in zones I or II. See introduction for changes to treatment approach following repair to tendons in digital zones III, IV, V, as well as for flexor pollicus longus.

SURGICAL AND TREATMENT PURPOSE

To restore maximum active flexor tendon gliding to assure effective finger joint motion. The two most common impediments to this goal are rupture of the tendon repair or scarring with adhesions. The surgical technique requires gentle tendon handling; strong, effective suture material with grasping stitches; and meticulous postoperative management. The zone of tendon injury may not coincide with the level of skin laceration due to finger position when the cut occurs. The zone within which

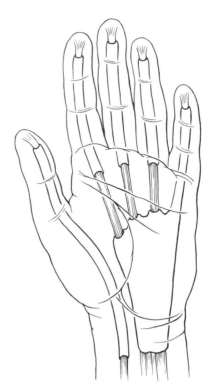

Fig. 11-1. Volar skin creases and their relationship to tendons in an extended position.

the tendon is repaired dictates to some extent the therapy methods to be used (Figs. 11-1 and 11-2). The thumb flexor tendon lies alone in the digital sheath whereas there are two intimately related tendons—profoundus and sublimis—in each digital sheath of the fingers. This fact will alter some of the therapy requirements for the fingers compared with those of the thumb. The causes of flexor tendon injury are most commonly traumatic; however, rheumatoid arthritis may also bring it about.

TREATMENT GOALS

    I. Prevent tendon rupture
   II. Prevent flexion contractures
  III. Promote tendon healing
  IV. Encourage tendon gliding
   V. Restore active range of motion (AROM) and passive range of motion (PROM)
  VI. Maintain full range of motion (ROM) of all uninvolved joints of affected upper extremity
 VII. Return to previous level of function

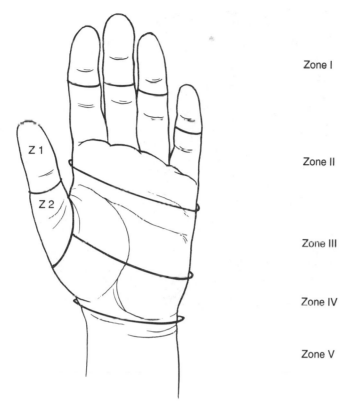

Zone I

Zone II

Zone III

Zone IV

Zone V

Fig. 11-2. Tendon zones.

POSTOPERATIVE INDICATIONS/PRECAUTIONS FOR THERAPY

I. Indications
    Surgical repair of flexor tendons to fingers and/or thumb
II. Precautions
    A. Infection
    B. Combined extensor tendon repair
    C. Fractures
    D. Nerve repair
    E. Vessel repair
    F. Extreme pain
    G. Severe edema

POSTOPERATIVE THERAPY

I. Immediately postoperative
    Dorsal plaster splint applied in the operating room with wrist in
    20 degrees to 30 degrees of flexion, metacarpophalangeal (MCP)

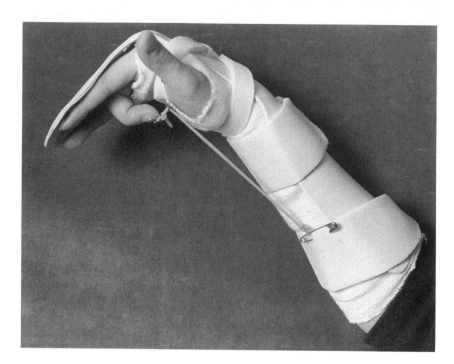

Fig. 11-3. Splinting with elastic traction to digital palmar crease and then to proximal forearm.

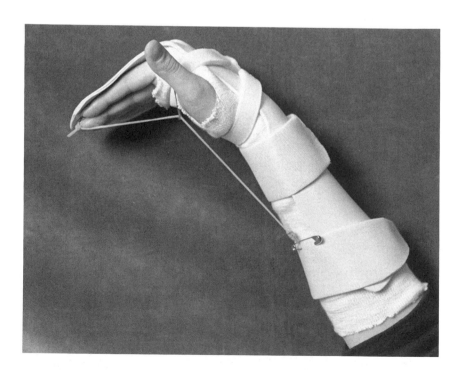

Fig. 11-4. Traction splint should allow full extension to limit of splint.

joints in 60 degrees to 70 degrees of flexion and full interphalangeal
(IP) joint extension.

II. 3 days postoperative
   A. Splint

      If cast is holding hand in proper position and is comfortable,
patient may remain in it. If not, a thermoplastic splint may be
fabricated dorsally with wrist at 20 degrees to 30 degrees of
flexion, MCP joints at 70 degrees flexion, allowing full IP joint
extension. Rubber band or elastic thread traction may be attached proximal to the wrist crease. The traction should allow
the finger to attain full active IP joint extension within cast or
splint limits and retain its natural alignment into flexion. An
alternate method of traction to the level of digital palmar crease
and then to proximal forearm may be used (Figs. 11-3 and 11-
4). If elastic traction is not used, digits may be maintained in
extension via Velcro strap to dorsum of splint. Strap is removed
for exercise.

   B. Exercise

      Active IP joint extension (with MCP joints passively flexed).
A proximal joint wedge that passively flexes MP joints may be
used to facilitate full proximal interphalangeal (PIP) joint extension. Passive flexion by isolating MCP joints, PIP joints, and
distal interphalangeal (DIP) joints, respectively. Passive composite flexion to the distal palmar crease and protected passive
extension.

   C. Edema control
   D. Pain control
   E. Wound care

III. 2 Weeks postoperative
   A. Wrist may be brought to neutral in splint.

IV. 3 weeks postoperative
   A. Tendon glide should be checked. If tendon becomes quickly
adherent, AROM into flexion may begin at 3 weeks. If early
tendon gliding is excellent, there are probably minimal adhesions. The tendon should be protected up to 2 to 3 weeks
longer.[4]

     1. Splint
       a. Continue as above.
     2. Exercise
       a. Progress from place and hold, to AROM (full fist/flat fist),
         to active blocked ROM.

V. 4 weeks postoperative.
   A. Splint
     1. Dorsal forearm based splint at night and in crowds or wristlet
       with rubber band traction worn at all times[3,4] (Fig. 11-5).
   B. Exercise
     1. Continue as above and add active hook fist and active MCP/

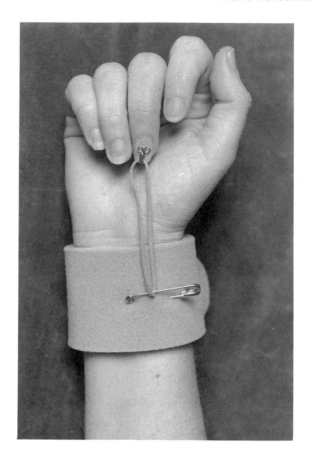

Fig. 11-5. Wristlet with rubber band traction.

   IP joint extension avoiding combined wrist and digit extension.
  C. Scar management
  D. Light activities of daily living (ADL)
VI. 6 weeks postoperative
  A. Splint
    1. Protective splint or wristlet discontinued[4]
    2. Gentle dynamic extension splinting to alleviate PIP joint contractures[4]
    3. Gentle progressive extension splint to control flexor tendon tightness
  B. Exercise
    1. Continue as above and for adherent tendons minimal resistance may be initiated with surgeon's approval.
VII. 8 weeks postoperative
  A. Progressive strengthening
  B. Graded work simulation may be initiated
VIII. 12 weeks postoperative
  A. Return to unrestricted activity

POSTOPERATIVE COMPLICATIONS

I. Tendon rupture
II. Minimal tendon gliding
III. Flexion contractures
IV. Excessive scar formation
V. Extreme pain
VI. Severe edema
VII. Infection

EVALUATION TIMELINE

I. First postoperative therapy session
   A. General assessment of
      1. Wound
      2. Edema
      3. Pain
      4. Sensibility
      5. Passive flexion and active PIP/DIP joint extension in protective splint
II. 6 weeks (or as early as 3 weeks with adherent tendons)
   A. AROM and PROM
III. 8 weeks
   A. Strength
IV. 12 weeks
   A. Heavy work assessment

REFERENCES

1. Duran RJ, Houser RG et al: Management of flexor tendon lacerations in zone 2 using controlled passive motion postoperatively. In Hunter JM, Schneider LH, Mackin EJ, Callahan AD (eds): Rehabilitation of the Hand. 2nd Ed. CV Mosby, St. Louis, 1984
2. Kleinert HE, Cash SL: Current guidelines for flexor tendon repair within the fibro-ossens tunnel: indications, timing and techniques. p. 117. In Hunter JM, Schneider LH, Mackin EJ (eds): Tendon Surgery in the Hand. CV Mosby, St. Louis, 1987
3. Cannon NM, Strickland JW: Therapy following flexor tendon surgery. Hand Clinics 1(1):147, 1985
4. Van Strien G: Postoperative management of flexor tendon injuries. In Hunter JM, Schneider LH, Mackin EJ, Callahan AD (eds): Rehabilitation of the Hand. 3rd Ed. CV Mosby, St. Louis, 1990

SUGGESTED READINGS

Amadio PS, Jaeger SH, Hunter JM: Nutritional aspects of tendon healing. In Hunter JM, Schneider LH, Mackin EJ, Callahan AD (eds): Rehabilitation of the Hand. 2nd Ed. CV Mosby, St. Louis, 1984

Cash SL: Primary care of flexor tendon injuries. In Hunter JM, Schneider LH, Mackin EJ, Callahan AD (eds): Rehabilitation of the Hand. 3rd Ed. CV Mosby, St. Louis, 1990

Chow JA, Thomas LJ et al: A combined regimen of controlled motion following flexor tendon repair in "No-Man's Land." J Plast Reconstr Surg 3(79):447, 1987

Creekmore H, Bellinghausen H et al: Comparison of early passive motion and immobilization after flexor tendon repairs. J Plast Reconstr Surg 1(75):75, 1985

Gelberman RH, Vandeberg JS et al: The early stages of flexor tendon healing: a morphological study of the first fourteen days. J Hand Surg (6)10A:776, 1985

Gelberman RH, Woo S et al: Effects of early passive mobilization on healing canine flexor tendons. J Hand Surg 7:170, 1982

Jaeger SH, Mackin EJ: Primary care of flexor tendon injuries. p. 261. In Hunter JM, Schneider LH, Mackin EJ, Callahan AD (eds): Rehabilitation of the Hand. 2nd Ed. CV Mosby, St. Louis, 1984

Kleinert HE, Kutz JE, Cohen MJ: Primary repair of zone 2 flexor tendon lacerations. p. 91. In: AAOS Symposium on Tendon Surgery in the Hand. CV Mosby, St. Louis, 1975

Kuxhaus M: Flexor and extensor repairs. In Ziegler EM (ed): Current Concepts in Orthotics—A Diagnosis Related Approach to Splinting. Roylan Medical Products, Menomonee Falls, 1984

Lister GD, Kleinert GE, Kutz JE et al: Primary flexor tendon repair followed by immediate controlled mobilization. J Hand Surg 2(6):441, 1977

Strickland JW: Results of flexor tendon surgery in zone II. Hand Clinics 1(1):167, 1985

Strickland JW: Biologic rationale, clinical application and results of early motion following flexor tendon repair. J Hand Ther 2(2):71, 1989

Flexor Tenolysis

12

Barbara Rabinowitz

Flexor tenolysis is an elective surgical procedure that may be performed status post primary tendon repair, grafting, or staged tendon reconstruction. It may be indicated when despite appropriate surgery and postoperative therapy with a highly motivated and compliant patient, active range of motion (AROM) is significantly less than passive range of motion (PROM) secondary to scar adhesions.[1]

Close surgeon–therapist communication is indicated prior to initiation of treatment to understand the condition of the tendon intraoperatively and to be made aware of any ancillary procedures. If the therapist is able to observe the surgery, this communication is greatly facilitated.

After surgery two different treatment approaches may be utilized for the first 4 to 6 weeks. Both approaches utilize early mobilization. With a good quality tendon and good quality pulleys (as noted by the surgeon intraoperatively), the more progressive approach may be utilized.[1,2] The "frayed tendon protocol"[1] is used with a poor quality tendon and/or after pulley reconstruction. If, while using the more progressive approach on an apparently good quality tendon without pulley reconstruction, an auditory or palpable crepitation is noted, it is important to move to the frayed tendon guideline as this may be a sign of impending rupture.[1] The frayed tendon guideline is used to decrease demands on the involved tendon or pulley while maintaining the tendon excursion achieved during surgery.

DEFINITION

Flexor tenolysis is a secondary surgical procedure in which adhesions or other obstacles that impede normal flexor tendon gliding are released (Fig. 12-1).

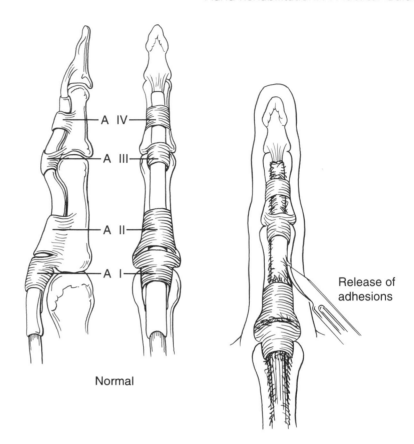

A IV

A III

A II

A I

Release of
adhesions

Normal

Fig. 12-1. Adhesions are released
in tenolysis surgery.

SURGICAL AND TREATMENT PURPOSE

To restore flexor tendon function to a finger or fingers when tendon gliding has been compromised or lost because of scar adhesions. The surgical approach may be very localized or very extensive depending on the preoperative as well as intraoperative assessment. Sharp dissection is used and great care is taken to preserve the critical portions of the digital pulley systems. Intraoperative assessment can be made by pulling on the tendons themselves or by carrying out the operation under local anesthesia in order that active motion can be observed. Early therapy is instituted on a very frequent basis to reduce the opportunities of re-scarring. Tendon rupture is a real and serious complication because tenolysis may render the structure avascular. Very careful and attentive postoperative care is required to achieve an optimal goal.

PURPOSE OF POSTOPERATIVE TREATMENT

   I. Maintain tendon excursion achieved intraoperatively
  II. Improve AROM and PROM
 III. Prevent tendon rupture

IV. Prevent flexion contracture
V. Protect repaired pulleys (if applicable)
VI. Modify pain
VII. Control edema
VIII. Maintain full range of motion (ROM) of all uninvolved joints of the affected upper extremity
IX. Return to previous level of function

POSTOPERATIVE INDICATIONS/PRECAUTIONS FOR THERAPY

I. Indications
    Digit(s) having undergone flexor tenolysis surgery
II. Precautions
    A. Pulley reconstruction
    B. Capsulectomy
    C. Poor quality or badly scarred tendon as reported by surgeon following procedure
    D. An auditory or palpable crepitation in the digit during early mobilization may indicate impending rupture

POSTOPERATIVE THERAPY

I. Consult with surgeon regarding
    A. Intraoperative ROM
    B. Condition of the tendon
    C. Status of the pulley system
    D. Additional procedures performed (i.e., pulley reconstruction or capsulectomy)
II. Pulley reconstruction protection[3]
    A. Identify areas of pulley reconstruction.
    B. Protect by circumferential taping or thermoplastic ring (Fig. 12-2).
    C. Continue protection 6 months postoperatively.
III. Capsulectomy
    A. See capsulectomy guideline.
    B. Treatment for tenolysis is determined by tendon quality.
IV. Program for good quality tendons
    A. 12 to 24 hours postoperative
        1. Splint
            a. Forearm based progressive extension or static extension[4] (Fig. 12-3) worn day and night for 2 weeks. Remove only for exercise and wound care.
        2. Exercise
            a. Active: 5 to 10 repetitions each exercise hourly.
                i. Place and hold as defined in Exercises Defined I.

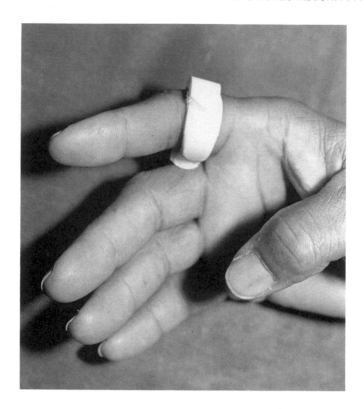

Fig. 12-2. Pulley reconstruction is protected by circumferential thermoplastic ring.

ii. Finger blocking as defined in Exercises Defined IV.
iii. Finger extension
   b. Passive: 5 to 10 repetitions three times per day[3,4] or as often as every hour if passive motion is limited.[1] Gentle, PROM all joints.
3. Edema control

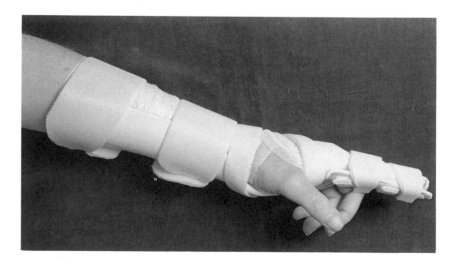

Fig. 12-3. A forearm based static extension splint is used postoperatively.

B. 2 weeks postoperative
1. Splint
   a. Static or progressive extension: decrease use in day as AROM achieved intraoperatively is maintained pain free. Continue use at night.
   b. Dynamic extension for contractures may be used with surgeon's approval, for short periods during the day (Fig. 12-4).
2. Exercise
   a. Continue exercises as above.
   b. Add active tendon gliding (3 to 10 repetitions per hour) as defined in Exercises Defined II.
3. Activities of daily living (ADL)
   a. Light ADL
   b. Grasp and release activities without resistance
   c. 4 to 7 weeks postoperative
      i. Splint
         A. Static or progressive extension. Wear in daytime only if needed. Continue night use for 6 months postoperatively.
         B. Dynamic extension
            If necessary to assist with extension, may leave on for most of the day. Patient may exercise into flexion against resistance of splint.

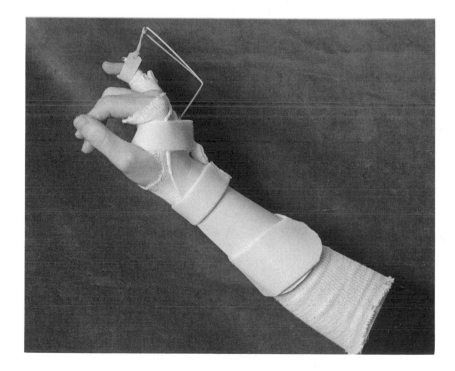

Fig. 12-4. Dynamic extension for contractures may be used with doctor's approval.

        ii. Exercise
          A. Continue exercises above as needed.
          B. Graded isometric grip strengthening with physician approval. Monitor closely.
       iii.
          A. ADL
          B. Graded ADL
    d. 8 to 12 weeks postoperative
      i. Gradually increase resistive exercises and activities to no restrictions at 12 weeks.

V. "Frayed tendon program"[1,2,5]
  A. Indications
    1. Surgical finding of poor quality tendon
    2. Pulleys reconstructed
    3. Tendons with auditory or palpable crepitation during uncomplicated early mobilization program
  B. First 4 to 6 weeks postoperative
    1. Splint: same as uncomplicated
    2. Exercise
      a. Protected PROM as defined in Exercises Defined III, 10 repetitions, three times daily
      b. Place and hold
  C. 7 to 12 weeks postoperative: see Postoperative Therapy IV

POSTOPERATIVE COMPLICATIONS

    I. Pain
   II. Edema
  III. Bleeding
 IV. Infection
   V. Patient's inability to tolerate postoperative therapy
 VI. Excessive scar formation
VII. Auditory or palpable crepitation
VIII. Tendon rupture
 IX. Flexion contractures
  X. Reconstructed pulley rupture
 XI. Minimal gain or actual loss of motion

EXERCISES DEFINED

  I. Place and hold technique[1]
    A. Passively manipulate the digit into the fully flexed position with the uninvolved hand.
    B. Patient actively maintains the digit in this position.
    C. Manipulation hand is released and lysed tendon(s) are maintained

in flexion with their own muscle power, confirming active muscle contraction. This is followed by actively extending the digit(s).

 D. Additional protection can be achieved by maintaining some element of wrist flexion although full excursion of tendon is not achieved in this position.

 E. The patient's discomfort level determines the beginning number of repetitions, maintaining frequency of every waking hour, working up to 10 repetitions per hour.

II. Tendon gliding technique as described by Wehbe[6]

 A. *Hook fist:* begin with the fingers in full extension. With metacarpophalangeal (MCP) joints in extension, actively flex proximal interphalangeal (PIP) joints and distal interphalangeal (DIP) joints. [Flexor digitorum superficialis (FDS) and flexor digitorum profundus (FDP) independently glide over each other most in this position.]

 B. *Full fist:* beginning in hook fist position, flex MCPs, PIPs, and DIPs fully, touching distal palmar crease. (FDP reaches its maximum excursion with respect to bone in this position.) End with fingers in full extension.

 C. *Straight fist:* begin with fingers in full extension. Actively flex MCPs and PIPs while maintaining DIPs in extension. (FDS reaches its maximum excursion in respect to bone in this position.)

III. Protected PROM technique

 Passively flex other digits and wrist while passively extending and flexing in turn the MCP, PIP, and DIP joints.

IV. Finger blocking technique

 A. Block MCP and PIP joints into extension, allowing isolated active DIP flexion.

 B. Block MCP into extension, allowing isolated PIP flexion.

EVALUATION TIMELINE

 I. 1 to 2 weeks preoperative
 A. AROM and PROM (blocked and full excursion)
 B. Fingertip to distal palmar crease (active and passive)
 C. Strength
 II. First postoperative therapy session (12 to 24 hours postoperative)
 A. Assessment
 1. Wound
 2. Edema
 3. Pain
 4. Sensibility
 B. Measurement
 1. AROM and PROM
 2. Fingertip to distal palmar crease (active and passive)
 III. ROM re-evaluated weekly first 8 weeks and then every 4 weeks

IV. Strength measurements at 8 weeks, then at 4-week intervals
V. Sensibility re-evaluated at 4 weeks, then at 4-week intervals

REFERENCES

1. Cannon NW, Strickland JW: Therapy following flexor tendon surgery. Hand Clinics 1(1):147, 1985
2. Strickland JW: Flexor tenolysis: a personal experience. p. 216. In Hunter JM, Schneider LH, Mackin EJ (eds): Tendon Surgery in the Hand. CV Mosby, St. Louis, 1987
3. Mackin EJ: Benefits of early tendon gliding after tenolysis. In Hunter JM, Schneider LH, Mackin EJ (eds): Tendon Surgery in the Hand. CV Mosby, St. Louis, 1987
4. Schneider LH, Mackin EJ: Tenolysis: dynamic approach to surgery and therapy. p. 417. In Hunter JM, Schneider LH, Mackin EJ, Callahan AD (eds): Rehabilitation of the Hand. 3rd Ed. CV Mosby, St. Louis, 1990
5. Strickland JW: Flexor tenolysis. Hand Clin 1(1):121, 1985
6. Wehbe MA: Tendon gliding exercises. Am J Occupat Ther 41(3):164, 1987

SUGGESTED READINGS

Cannon NW: Enhancing flexor tendon glide through tenolysis . . . and hand therapy. J Hand Ther 2(2):122, 1989
Schneider LH: Flexor tenolysis. In Hunter JM, Schneider LH, Mackin EJ (eds): Tendon Surgery in the Hand. CV Mosby, St. Louis, 1987
Verdan C: Tenolysis: p. 137. In Verdan C (ed): Tendon Surgery of the Hand. Churchill Livingstone, New York, 1979

Primary Tendon Grafts

13

Barbara Rabinowitz

Although primary flexor tendon repair is generally the best postinjury treatment choice, there are times when this is neither possible nor indicated. These include, but are not limited to, the following situations: the wound or the patient's general condition may disallow direct repair,[1] a flexor tendon injury may be missed at the time of injury,[1] or there may be a late referral for definitive care that may make it impossible for the surgeon to perform an end to end repair.[1]

Three basic postsurgical treatment approaches are described below. The first is early mobilization similar to zone II primary flexor tendon repairs.[2] The second is 3 to 4 weeks immobilization.[2] The third is the situation in which the flexor digitorum profundus is repaired in a digit with a noninjured flexor digitorum superficialis.[3]

As with primary tendon repairs, it is necessary to adjust the progression of treatment according to the "feel" of the tendon graft as it is healing. When early recovery of active range of motion (AROM) is seen and the tendon is gliding well, protective splinting is continued longer and treatment progresses more slowly as the risk of tendon rupture is greater in the "soft healers."[1]

Conversely, where little active tendon glide is noted when AROM is initiated, progression may need to be faster (in consultation with physician) to decrease the effect of tendon adhesions while preventing tendon rupture.

Judgement must also be used in educating the more active or impulsive patient as well as the more reluctant to facilitate patient compliance in achieving the best result with the fewest complications.

DEFINITION

Removal of injured tendon and replacement with palm to fingertip tendon graft (Fig. 13-1)

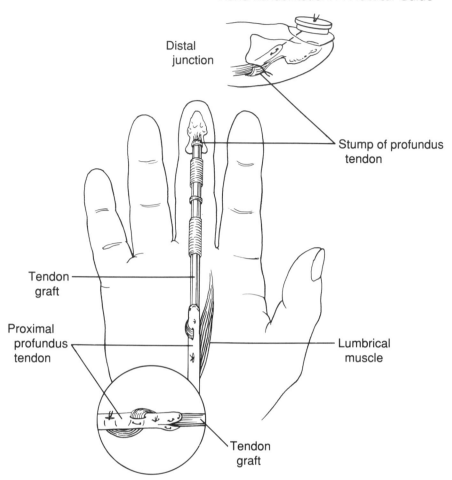

Fig. 13-1. Injured tendon is removed and replaced with a tendon graft.

SURGICAL PURPOSE

Following flexor or extensor tendon injuries or conditions that cause scarring that prevents tendon gliding, tendon grafting is sometimes indicated. The tendon graft is used to bridge a gap between the muscle unit and the insertion of the tendon into bone. It is most commonly employed for the flexor tendons that have been interrupted between the origin of the lumbrical muscles and their distal insertion.

TREATMENT GOALS

I. Loss of both flexor digitorum superficialis (FDS)/flexor digitorum profundus (FDP) function
   A. Preoperative
      1. Full passive range of motion (PROM) proximal interphalangeal (PIP) and distal interphalangeal (DIP) joints
      2. Soft, pliable tissues

   3. Patient education regarding
      a. Preoperative therapy
      b. Postoperative therapy
   B. Postoperative
      1. Prevent rupture at proximal and distal tendon junctures.
      2. Minimize adhesion formation.
      3. Prevent flexion contractures.
      4. Prevent hyperextension deformity at PIP joint, which can occur
         with absent superficialis.
      5. Promote tendon healing.
      6. Encourage tendon gliding.
      7. Restore AROM and PROM.
      8. Maintain full AROM of all uninvolved joints of affected upper
         extremity.
      9. Return to previous level of function.
II. FDS intact/FDP absent.
    Pre- and post-operative goals are the same as above, except add
   A. Preoperative: normal FDS AROM and PROM.
   B. Postoperative: regain active superficialis function while protecting
      profundus graft.

PREOPERATIVE INDICATIONS FOR THERAPY

I. Indications
   A. Decreased range of motion (ROM)
   B. Adherent scar
   C. Weak proximal muscle units

PREOPERATIVE THERAPY

  I. Patient education regarding complexity of rehabilitation and neces-
     sary patient compliance
 II. Scar management
III. PROM
IV. AROM of PIP joint if FDS uninvolved
 V. Strengthening
    A. Proximal flexor motor units
    B. Extrinsic/intrinsic extensors

POSTOPERATIVE INDICATIONS/PRECAUTIONS
FOR THERAPY

I. Indications
   Digit has undergone free tendon grafting procedure.

II. Precautions
  A. Avoid strengthening until 9 to 10 weeks following graft due to avascular nature of free tendon grafts.[2]
  B. Protect reconstructed pulleys if indicated.

POSTOPERATIVE THERAPY

I. Both FDS/FDP absent preoperatively
  A. Two approaches
    1. Early mobilization
      a. Weeks 0 to 8: same as zone II flexor tendon guideline except delay in strengthening.
      b. Weeks 9 to 10: initiate graded strengthening.
      c. Weeks 12 to 14: normal unrestricted use of hand.
    2. Early immobilization
      a. Weeks 0 to 3 or 4
          Splint: posterior plaster or thermoplastic with wrist 20 degrees to 30 degrees flexion, MCP joints 60 degrees to 70 degrees of flexion and IP joints in extension.
      b. Weeks 3 to 4
        i. Splint: worn between exercise programs for 1 to 2 additional weeks.
        ii. Exercise: AROM initiated.
      c. Weeks 4 to 14: same as early mobilization
II. FDS intact with FDP absent preoperatively[3]
    Weeks 0 to 8: same as above (Postoperative Therapy I) except active isolated FDS flexion begun at week 1 with wrist and MCPs flexed while holding unaffected digits (PIPs/DIPs) in passive extension.

POSTOPERATIVE COMPLICATIONS

  I. Tendon rupture
  II. Adhesions limiting tendon gliding
  III. Flexion contracture
  IV. Extreme pain
  V. Severe edema
  VI. Infection
  VII. Pulley ruptured or attenuated
  VIII. Suboptimal graft length

EVALUATION TIME LINE

  I. Preoperative
    A. Wound and skin condition
    B. Edema

- C. Pain
- D. Sensibility
- E. PROM
- F. AROM
- G. Strength
II. Postoperative
- A. First postoperative visit gross assessment of:
    1. Wound and skin condition
    2. Edema
    3. Pain
    4. Sensibility
    5. Passive flexion
- B. Week 6: active and passive motion
- C. Week 12: Strength

REFERENCES

1. Schneider LH, Hunter JM: Flexor tendons—late reconstruction. p. 1969. In Green DP (ed): Operative Hand Surgery. Vol. 3. Churchill Livingstone, New York, 1988
2. Cannon NM: Therapy following flexor tendon surgery. p. 147. Hand Clinics 1(1):156, 1985
3. McClinton MA, Curtis RM, Wilgis EFS: One hundred tendon grafts for isolated flexor digitorum injuries. J Hand Surg 7(3):224, 1982

Staged Tendon Reconstruction

14

Barbara Rabinowitz

Staged tendon reconstruction is a salvage procedure. Therapy for this procedure consists of three parts: preoperative, postoperative stage I, and postoperative stage II.

At the preoperative phase, patient education is a major component. The purpose of patient education is twofold. The first is to educate the patient regarding the surgical and rehabilitative requirements of these procedures. The second purpose of patient education is to monitor the patient's compliance with preoperative therapy to help assess the patient's willingness and ability to follow through with postoperative therapy.

Therapist–surgeon communication regarding surgical details is indicated after stage I and II procedures. After stage I, the therapist should be made aware of any other procedures such as pulley reconstruction or joint releases. After stage II, the therapist should be made aware of the amount of tension on the graft and the predicted active motion of the digit.

DEFINITION

Staged tendon reconstruction is a two-stage tendon graft procedure with implantation of Silastic rod at stage I to establish a smooth walled channel.[1,2] This is followed by removal of the implant and placement of a free tendon graft within the neosheath at stage II[1-3] (Figs. 14-1 and 14-2).

SURGICAL PURPOSE

Staged tendon reconstruction is employed most often for the flexor units although the technique may be used for the extensors. It is utilized when there is a scarred bed through which the tendons may be required to

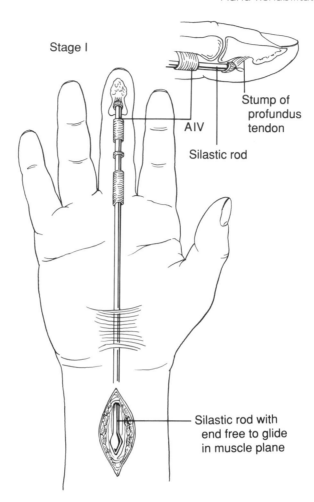

Stage I

Stump of
profundus
tendon

AIV

Silastic rod

Silastic rod with
end free to glide
in muscle plane

Fig. 14-1. Digit with silastic rod during stage I.

glide. Concomitantly pulley reconstructions may be necessary. A passive tendon prosthesis of silicone is placed in the finger and palm to create a new tendon sheath through which an autologous tendon is passed later. The method is primarily used for salvage operations when other alternatives are not available.

TREATMENT GOALS

I. Preoperative
   A. Restoration of passive range of motion (PROM) with fingertip passively touching distal palmar crease.
   B. Maintain or re-establish supple soft tissues.
   C. Maintain or re-establish strength of proximal muscles.
   D. Promote balanced flexion–extension system.
II. Postoperative stage I
   A. Continue with goals A through D above.

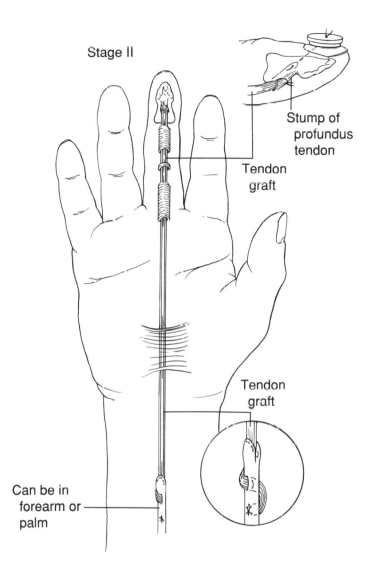

Stage II

Stump of
profundus
tendon

Tendon
graft

Tendon
graft

Can be in
forearm or
palm

Fig. 14-2. Digit with graft within neosheath at stage II.

    B. Facilitate proximal portion of sheath formation in as lengthened
       a position as possible via splinting.[4]
III. Postoperative stage II
    A. Prevent rupture at proximal and distal tendon junctures.
    B. Minimize adhesion formation.
    C. Prevent flexion contractures.
    D. Prevent hyperextension deformity at proximal interphalangeal
       (PIP) joint, which can occur with absent superficialis.
    E. Promote tendon healing.
    F. Encourage tendon gliding.
    G. Restore active range of motion (AROM) and passive range of mo-
       tion (PROM).

   H. Maintain full AROM of all uninvolved joints of affected upper extremity.
    I. Return to previous level of function.

INDICATIONS FOR PREOPERATIVE THERAPY

   I. Decreased range of motion (ROM)
  II. Adherent scar
 III. Weak proximal muscle units

PREOPERATIVE THERAPY

   I. Exercise
    A. PROM
    B. "Finger trapping"[2]
  II. Splinting
    A. Flexion limited
      1. Buddy taping (Fig. 14-3).
      2. Intrinsic stretch splinting (Fig. 14-4)
      3. PIP/distal interphalangeal (DIP) joint flexion straps (Fig. 14-5)
    B. Extension limited
      1. Three-point extension splint (Fig. 14-6)

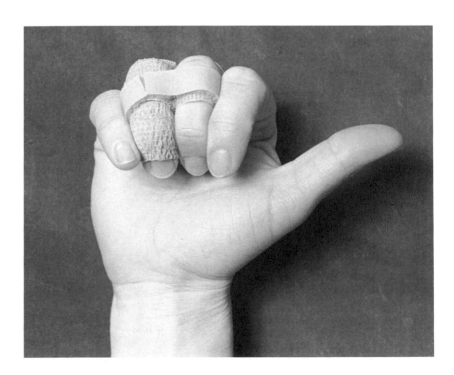

Fig. 14-3. Buddy taping to facilitate increased flexion.

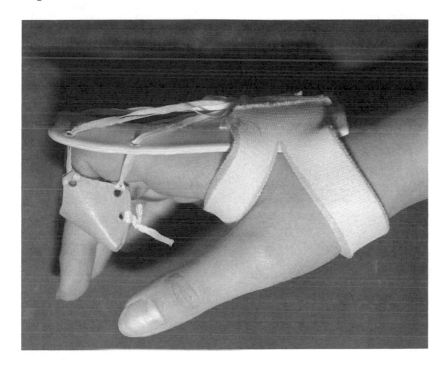

Fig. 14-4. Intrinsic stretch splinting to increase flexion.

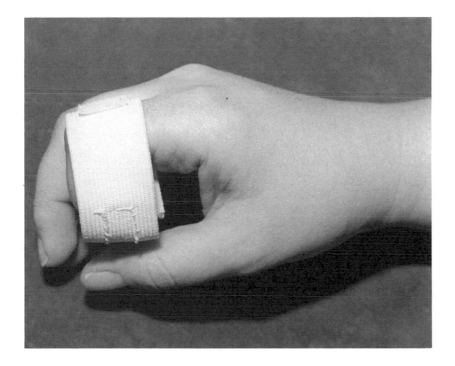

Fig. 14-5. PIP/DIP flexion strap for improving flexion.

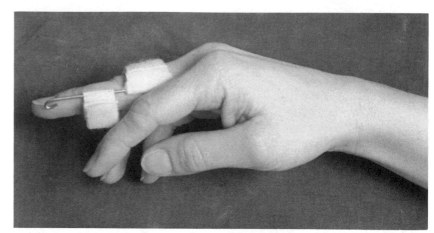

Fig. 14-6. Three-point extension splint to increase extension.

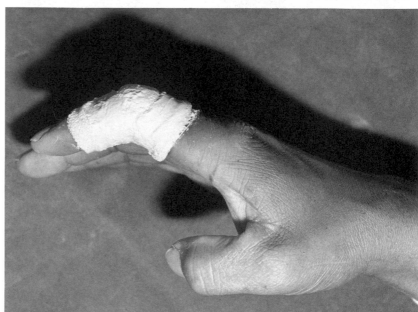

Fig. 14-7. Serial casts can help increase extension.

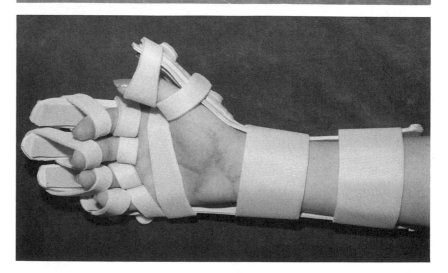

Fig. 14-8. Serially applied thermoplastic splints can increase extension.

      2. Serial casts (Fig. 14-7)
      3. Serially applied thermoplastic splints (Fig. 14-8)
III. Strengthening

INDICATIONS/PRECAUTIONS FOR
POSTOPERATIVE THERAPY

I. Indications
      Digit has undergone stage I or stage II tendon reconstruction.
II. Precautions
   A. Stage I postoperative
      1. Avoid overexercising, which can lead to synovitis.
      2. Avoid attenuation of extensor tendon at DIP joint.
      3. Protect reconstructed pulleys if present.
   B. Stage II postoperative
      Monitor pain at insertion, which could be precursor of rupture.

POSTOPERATIVE THERAPY

I. Stage I
   A. Immediately postoperative
      Splint: dorsal protective splint with wrist in 30 degrees flexion,
      metacarpophalangeal (MCP) joints in 60 degrees to 70 degrees
      flexion, and interphalangeal (IP) joints in full extension (Fig. 14-
      9).
   B. Day 1 to 3 weeks postoperative
      1. PROM
      2. Wound care
      3. Edema control
      4. Scar management
   C. 3 weeks to 6 weeks
      1. Splint
         a. Protective splint discontinued unless signs of synovitis are
            present.
         b. Initiate splints to facilitate full PROM.
         c. Figure-of-eight splint for PIP joint if "swan-neck" deformity
            is present or developing (Fig. 14-10). Continue until volar
            plate is strong enough to support PIP joint or until stage II
            surgery is performed.[4]
      2. Exercise, wound care, edema control, and scar management
         continue.
   D. 6 weeks
      1. Return to normal activities.
      2. Treatment continued until stage I goals are met.

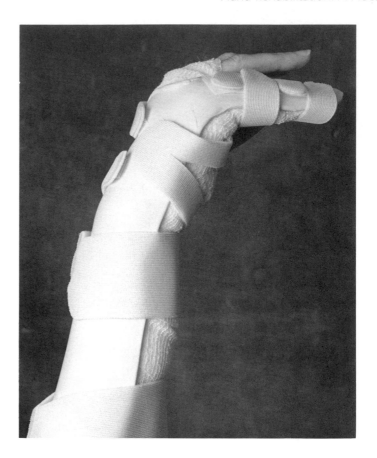

Fig. 14-9. Dorsal protective splint following stage I surgery.

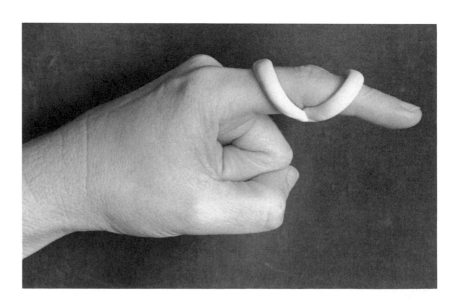

Fig. 14-10. Figure of eight splint is used if "swan-neck" deformity is present or develops.

II. Stage II

Same as zone II primary flexor tendon graft: see appropriate guideline.

POSTOPERATIVE COMPLICATIONS

I. Stage I
- A. Synovitis
- B. Swan-neck deformity
- C. Limited ROM/attenuation of extensor tendon
- D. Skin breakdown at distal insertion of implant
- E. Implant "kinking" or disruption
- F. Pain
- G. Edema
- H. Hematoma
- I. Infection

II. Stage II
- A. Tendon rupture
- B. Adhesions limiting tendon gliding
- C. Flexion contracture
- D. Extreme pain
- E. Severe edema
- F. Infection
- G. Suboptimal graft length

EVALUATION TIMELINE

I. Preoperative
- A. Wound and skin condition
- B. Edema
- C. Pain
- D. Sensibility
- E. PROM
- F. AROM
- G. Strength

II. Stage I postoperative
- A. Wound
- B. Edema
- C. Pain
- D. Sensibility
- E. Passive flexion
- F. Active PIP/DIP extension with wrist and MCP flexed

III. Stage II postoperative
- A. First postoperative visit general assessment of
  1. Wound and skin condition
  2. Edema

3. Pain
4. Sensibility
5. Passive flexion/protected active/passive extension
B. Week 6: active flexion and passive extension
C. Week 12: strength

REFERENCES

1. Cannon NM, Strickland JW: Therapy following flexor tendon surgery. Hand Clinics 1(1):156, 1985
2. Mackin EJ, Hunter JM: Pre- and Post-Operative Hand Therapy Program for Patients with Staged Tendon Implants (Hunter Design). Hand Rehabilitation Foundation, Philadelphia, 1986
3. Hunter JM, Singer DI, Mackin EJ: Staged flexor tendon reconstruction using passive and active tendon implants. p. 427. In Hunter JM, Schneider LH, Mackin EJ, Callahan AD (eds): Rehabilitation of the Hand, 3rd Ed. CV Mosby, St. Louis, 1990
4. Stanley BG: Flexor tendon injuries: late solution therapist's management. Hand Clin 12(1):140, 1986

SUGGESTED READINGS

Hunter JM, Blackmore SM, Callahan AD: Flexor tendon salvage and functional redemption using the Hunter tendon implant and the superficialis Finer operation. J Hand Ther 2(2):107, 1989
Hunter JM, Daniel IS, Jaeger SH et al: Active tendon implants in flexor tendon reconstruction. J Hand Surg 13A(6):849, 1988
Lister MBG: Pitfalls and complications of flexor tendon surgery. Hand Clinics 1(1):133, 1985
Schneider LH, Hunter JM: Flexor tendons—late reconstruction. p. 1967. In Green DP (ed): Operative Hand Surgery. Vol. 3. Churchill Livingstone, New York, 1988
Wehbe MA: Staged tendon reconstruction: technique and repair. p. 260. In Hunter JM, Schneider LH, Mackin EJ (eds): Tendon Surgery in the Hand. CV Mosby, St. Louis, 1987
Wehbe MA: Tendon gliding exercises. Am J Occupat Ther 41(3):164, 1987

Mallet Finger   **15**

Arlynne Pack Brown

Mallet finger injury is a traumatic disruption of the terminal tendon resulting in a loss of active extension of the distal interphalangeal (DIP) joint. This may or may not be associated with a fracture of the articular surface. Names synonymous with mallet finger injury are baseball finger[1] and drop finger.[2]

The primary goal of rehabilitation is to promote healing of the tendon so as to maximize function and range of motion (ROM) of the injured DIP joint.

Ruptures and lacerations may be treated closed with noninvasive splint immobilization or open with Kirschner wire (K-wire) fixation. Avulsion fractures are commonly secured into bone using the button technique with interosseus wire.

Whether immobilized closed with splints or open with K-wires or the button technique, the first 6 weeks of treatment are the same. During this initial period, the involved joint is immobilized full time while exercises are performed to maintain the ROM of the uninvolved joints. At the conclusion of the initial immobilization, the splints or internal fixators are removed and the integrity of the terminal tendon evaluated. If the tendon is unable to maintain extension and the joint droops into flexion, a splint is reapplied and tested periodically thereafter for healing and strength. When the tendon is "healed" enough, active flexion and extension is begun, monitored for overstretching, and progressed or digressed in ROM and strengthening exercises as indicated.

DEFINITION

I. Traumatically induced loss of active extension of the DIP joint caused by avulsion, rupture, laceration of the terminal tendon,[3] or fractured base of distal phalanx with tendon insertion attached (Fig. 15-1).

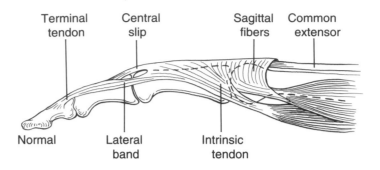

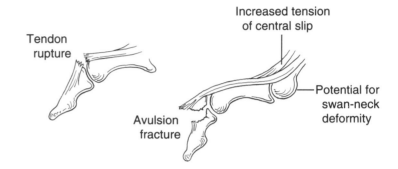

Fig. 15-1. Normal anatomy and two variations of mallet finger injury.

II. Injury may be classified according to the amount of articular surface involved in the associated fracture.[4]
   A. Type A: fracture of less than one-third of the articular surface
   B. Type B: fracture of one-third to two-thirds of the articular surface
   C. Type C: fracture of greater than two-thirds of the articular surface
   D. Note additional category of fracture dislocation DIP joint.
III. Other names for mallet finger injury
   A. Mallet finger deformity[3]
   B. Baseball finger[1]
   C. Drop finger[2]

TREATMENT AND SURGICAL PURPOSE

To restore extension to the DIP joint where there has been disruption of the terminal portion of the extensor tendon. When the injury is closed and the tendon continuity is lost, splinting of the DIP joint is preferred. If there has been a laceration of the tendon, a surgical repair by suture may be indicated. An avulsion fracture of the distal phalanx without DIP dislocation may be treated by splinting with the joint in extension. When there is an avulsion fracture with volar subluxation of the distal phalanx, open reduction and internal fixation is considered. The results of the foregoing treatment regimen frequently provide a good result; however, a permanent extension lag at the DIP joint may be anticipated. In some patients a concurrent hyperextension posture of the proximal interphalangeal (PIP) joint can be noted.

TREATMENT GOALS

I. Promote healing of terminal tendon and associated fracture.
II. Maintain full ROM of all uninvolved joints of the upper extremity.
III. Prevent swan-neck deformity and DIP joint flexion contracture.
IV. Avoid pin tract infection if applicable.
V. Maximize ROM of DIP joint and PIP joint. In particular, maximize active DIP joint extension.
VI. Return to previous level of function.
VII. Prevent re-injury.

NONOPERATIVE INDICATIONS/PRECAUTIONS FOR THERAPY

I. Indications
    A. Mallet finger injury without fracture
    B. Mallet finger injury associated with nondisplaced fracture
II. Precautions
    A. Extreme pain
    B. Extreme edema
    C. Tape allergy[5]

NONOPERATIVE THERAPY

I. Management of closed treatment
    A. Weeks 0 to 6: continuous splinting in 0 degrees or slight hyperextension (see Splints below). Change adhesive tape and check skin regularly.
    B. Weeks 6 to 7: Continue day and night splint. Begin active flexion up to 20 degrees to 25 degrees.[6] May use a volar template to limit flexion during exercise.
    C. Weeks 7 to 8: Continue day and night splint. If no extension lag, begin active flexion to 35 degrees.[6]
    D. Weeks 8 to 12: If no extension lag, discontinue day splint but continue night splint. If extension lag persists, balance splinting and exercise to minimize lag.
    E. Week 12: begin unrestricted use.
II. Splints[5-8]
    A. Position DIP joint at 0 degrees or slight hyperextension. Hyperextend DIP joint without blanching dorsal skin.[2,6]

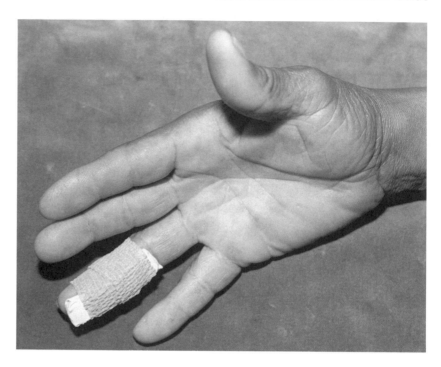

Fig. 15-2. Alumifoam splint.

B. Splints may be on dorsal or volar surface.
   1. Dorsal
      a. Advantages: does not interfere with PIP joint flexion; allows
         for sensibility of tip.
C. Splint types
   1. Alumifoam (Fig. 15-2)
   2. Stack (Fig. 15-3)

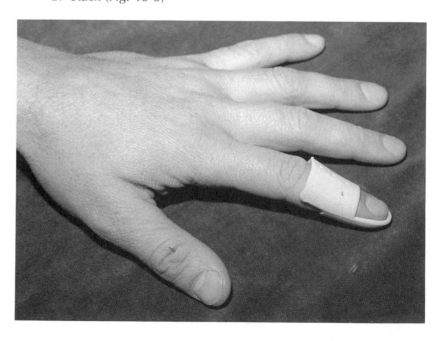

Fig. 15-3. Stack splint.

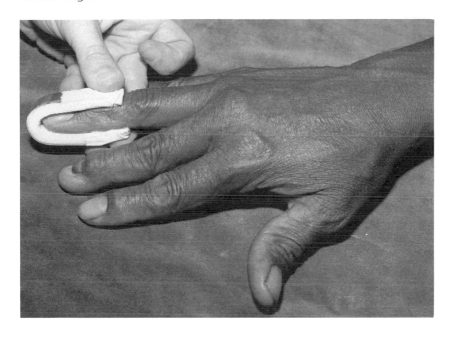

Fig. 15-4. Sugar tong alumifoam splint.

3. Sugar tong alumifoam (Fig. 15-4)
4. Custom thermoplastic (Fig. 15-5)
D. Splint fasteners
  1. Adhesive tape
  2. Velcro: may not provide enough security against axial rotation and distal slippage of splint
  3. Coban

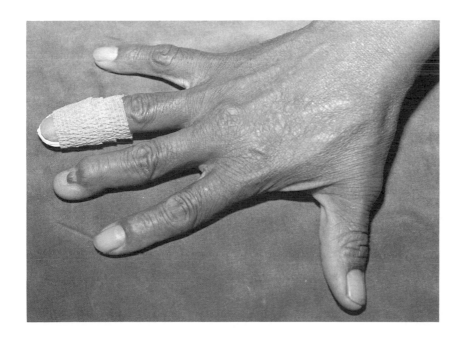

Fig. 15-5. Custom thermoplastic splint.

NONOPERATIVE COMPLICATIONS

   I. Maceration or necrosis of skin[4,5,7]
  II. Maceration or necrosis of nailbed[7]
 III. Swan-neck deformity[4]
 IV. Tape allergy[5]
  V. Extension lag at DIP joint[2]

POSTOPERATIVE INDICATIONS/PRECAUTIONS FOR THERAPY

   I. Indications
      Avulsions, ruptures, or lacerations of the terminal tendon with associated intra-articular DIP joint fractures managed with K-wires or buttons
  II. Precautions
    A. Infection
    B. Extreme pain
    C. Extreme edema

POSTOPERATIVE THERAPY

   I. Week 0 to 6
    A. K-wire or button intact
    B. ROM of uninvolved joints
    C. Pin site care
  II. Week 6
    A. K-wire removed.
    B. Begin active ROM (AROM) and follow closed treatment as described above.

POSTOPERATIVE COMPLICATIONS

   I. Infection
  II. Necrosis of nailbed[7]
 III. DIP joint extension lag
 IV. Swan-neck deformity[4]

EVALUATION TIMELINE

   I. Week 1
    A. AROM and passive ROM (PROM) of all upper extremity joints except involved DIP joint
    B. Sensibility

II. Week 6
   Active extensive DIP joint
III. Week 8
   Active flexion DIP joint
IV. Week 10
   A. Grip and pinch strength
   B. Passive flexion at DIP joint

REFERENCES

1. Wilson RL: Management of acute extensor tendon injuries. p. 337. In Hunter JM, Schneider LH, Mackin EJ (eds): Tendon Surgery of the Hand. CV Mosby, St. Louis, 1987
2. Clement RC, Wray RC: Operative and nonoperative treatment of mallet finger. Ann Plast Surg 1b:136, 1986
3. Elliott RA: Splints for mallet and boutonniere deformities. Plast Reconstr Surg 52:282, 1973
4. Wehbe MA, Schneider LH: Mallet fractures. J Bone Joint Surg 66:658, 1984
5. Stern PJ: Complications and prognosis of treatment of mallet finger. J Hand Surg. 13A:329, 1988
6. Evans RE: Therapeutic management of extensor tendon injuries. p. 492. In Hunter JM, Schneider LH, Mackin EJ, Callahan AD (eds): Rehabilitation of the Hand. CV Mosby, Baltimore, 1990
7. Hunter JM, Schneider LH, Mackin EJ, Callahan AD (eds): Rehabilitation of the Hand. CV Mosby, Baltimore, 1990
8. Patel MR, DeSai SS, Bassini-Lipson L: Conservative management of chronic mallet finger. J Hand Surg 11A:570, 1986

Swan-neck Deformity 16

Dale Eckhaus

Swan-neck deformities occur through extrinsic, intrinsic, and articular abnormal anatomical factors.[1] The etiology of these factors include: rheumatologic disease, extensor terminal tendon injuries, spastic conditions, injuries that cause volar plate laxity, fractures to the middle phalanx that heal in hyperextension, and generalized ligamentous laxity.[2] The deformity may also occur secondary to surgical procedures such as a flexor digitorum profundus (FDP) graft where the flexor digitorum superficialis (FDS) is absent. The deformity is one in which function decreases as the proximal interphalangeal (PIP) joint loses its flexibility. The lateral bands become dorsally displaced and tension to extend the distal interphalangeal (DIP) joint is reduced (Fig. 16-1). Treatment of the condition depends upon the etiologic status of the PIP joint and its related anatomic structures. Classification of the deformity may help determine treatment method. Four classifications have been described as follows: (1) PIP flexion remains supple in all positions, (2) PIP flexion is limited by intrinsic tightness, (3) PIP flexion is limited in all positions by articular factors and the joint remains good radiographically, (4) PIP flexion is limited in all positions by intra-articular factors as noted radiographically.[3]

Successful treatment of swan-neck deformity is dependent upon careful examination and determination of contributing factors.

DEFINITION

Deformity in which the PIP joint is hyperextended and the DIP joint is flexed (Fig. 16-2).

137

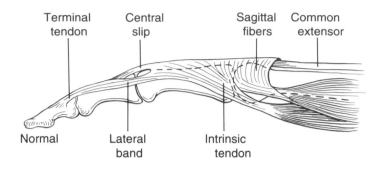

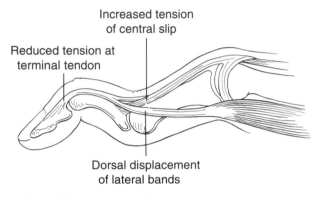

Fig. 16-1. Normal finger anatomy/dorsal subluxation of the lateral bands.

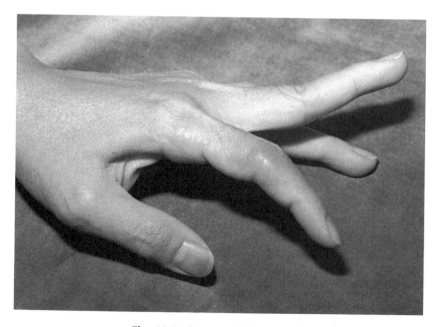

Fig. 16-2. Swan-neck deformity.

SURGICAL PURPOSE

To prevent hyperextension posture of the PIP joint with accompanying flexion of the DIP joint. Nonoperative splinting may be used temporarily to restore extensor tendon balance and to prevent fixed contractures. Surgical correction may be obtained by tendon transfers for active dynamic restoration of this balance. Such transfers may involve using the superficialis tendons of a wrist extensor prolonged with tendon grafts into the extensor mechanism. The passive restoration of balance includes a tenodesis of the PIP joint using local tendons or using a tendon graft to bridge the PIP joint.

TREATMENT GOALS

I. Nonoperative
   A. Promote balance of the extensor mechanism.
   B. Reduce intrinsic tightness.
   C. Maximize joint range of motion (ROM).
   D. Maintain ROM of wrist and uninvolved digits.
II. Postoperative
   A. Promote wound healing.
   B. Control edema.
   C. Control scar formation.
   D. Prevent attenuation or rupture of surgical procedure.
   E. Limit PIP extension and encourage full DIP extension.
   F. Promote full active flexion.
   G. Maintain ROM of uninvolved digits.

NONOPERATIVE INDICATIONS/PRECAUTIONS FOR THERAPY

I. Indications
   Supple deformities where prevention of PIP hyperextension restores DIP extension
II. Precautions
   A. Volar plate laxity
   B. Intrinsic tightness
   C. Dynamic imbalance originating at other joints or due to systemic or neurologic conditions

NONOPERATIVE THERAPY

I. Active and passive joint ROM
II. Intrinsic stretch exercises
III. Splint to balance finger extension. A tri-point splint prevents PIP joint hyperextension and restores DIP joint extension. This type of splint

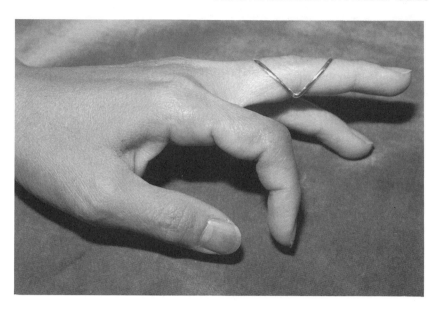

Fig. 16-3. Tri-point splint.

places dorsal pressure proximal and distal to the PIP joint and volar pressure at the PIP joint. It allows full active flexion (Fig. 16-3).

POSTOPERATIVE INDICATIONS/PRECAUTIONS FOR THERAPY

I. Indications
   A. Following surgical procedures designed to relieve the deformity
II. Precautions
   A. Excessive exercise that could cause attenuation or rupture of tenodesis procedures
   B. Procedures that involve joint fusions
   C. Procedures involving joint arthroplasty
   D. Surgical treatment requiring capsulectomy
   E. Surgical treatment requiring tenolysis
   F. Procedure requiring intrinsic release or metacarpophalangeal (MCP) joint surgical treatment

POSTOPERATIVE THERAPY

I. General care
   A. Edema control
   B. Wound care
   C. Scar management

    D. Pain management

    E. Maintain ROM of uninvolved digits

II. Treatment following tenodesis procedures of PIP joint

    A. Immediately postoperative wrist is splinted in slight extension[1] with MCP joint in slight flexion. The PIP joint is held in 20 degrees to 30 degrees of flexion and the DIP joint is positioned at 0 degrees.

    B. Active motion allowing full flexion and limiting extension of PIP 20 degrees to 30 degrees begins 1 to 4 weeks postoperative.[1-3] A Kirschner wire (K-wire) or splint may be used to hold DIP in extension in order that maximal flexion occurs at PIP joint.[1] Extension splint for DIP joint can continue for 6 weeks postoperative.

    C. Forearm based splint is replaced at 3 to 4 weeks by a hand based splint that allows ROM as noted above.

    D. Splinting to improve PIP flexion may be initiated if necessary at 3 weeks postoperative.

    E. At 6 to 10 weeks postoperative, PIP joint extension is permitted to gradually increase. Splint is adjusted to allow increased active extension or patient is permitted to decrease use of splint. Passive extension exercises for PIP joint are rarely necessary. PIP joint extension increases gradually over several months. A slight limitation in PIP extension is acceptable and expected. Dynamic extension splinting may be initiated at 6 weeks for PIP extension limitation greater than 20 degrees. Strengthening for flexion may begin at 6 weeks.

III. Other procedures

    Swan-neck deformity in rheumatoid arthritis commonly requires treatment by PIP joint arthroplasty. Details concerning the rehabilitation of this procedure are noted in the appropriate guideline.

COMPLICATIONS

I. Nonoperative

    A. Continuation of deformity

    B. Reducible deformity becomes fixed

    C. Reduction of hand function

II. Operative

    A. Infection

    B. Excessive edema

    C. Pain

    D. Rupture of tenodesis

    E. Attenuation of tenodesis

    F. Excessive scarring

    G. Limited ROM

EVALUATION TIMELINE

I. Nonoperative
   A. Initial evaluation
      1. Active ROM (AROM) and passive ROM (PROM): determine limiting factors if present.
      2. Strength
   B. Re-evaluate in 4 weeks.
II. Operative: following tenodesis procedures
   A. Initial postoperative visit
      1. Condition of surgical sites
      2. Edema
      3. Sensation
      4. Pain
      5. Management of activities of daily living (ADL)
   B. Weeks 1 to 4
      1. Active flexion and extension to limit of splint
      2. Passive flexion of PIP joint and MCP joint
   C. Week 6
      1. Passive flexion and extension all joints
      2. Grip strength/pinch strength

REFERENCES

1. Tubiana R: The swan neck deformity. p. III:125. In Tubiana R (ed): The Hand. Vol. III. WB Saunders, Philadelphia, 1988
2. Burton RI: Extensor tendons—late reconstruction. p. III:2073. In Green DP (ed): Operative Hand Surgery. 2nd Ed. Vol. 3. Churchill Livingstone, New York, 1988
3. Nalebuff EA: The rheumatoid swan neck deformity. p. V:203. In Feldon P: Rheumatoid Arthritis. In Peterson BL (ed): Hand Clinics. Vol. 5. WB Saunders, Philadelphia, 1989

Boutonnière Deformity　17

Lauren Valdata Eddington

The boutonnière or "buttonhole" deformity occurs when the common extensor tendon that inserts on the base of the middle phalanx is damaged and a volar sliding or subluxation of the lateral extensor bands occurs. These lateral extensor bands sublux volarly to the axis of the proximal interphalangeal (PIP) joint when the spiral fibers and transverse fibers are ruptured. The PIP joint then herniates, forms a buttonhole, and assumes a flexed position. With progression of the deformity, proximal retraction of the extensor apparatus will occur; this can put the metacarpophalangeal (MP) joint into hyperextension. The distal phalanx is also involved when the oblique retinacular ligament contracts and the distal phalanx is held in hyperextension[1-3] (Fig. 17-1).

The boutonnière deformity can result from injuries caused by division, rupture, avulsion, laceration, or closed trauma to the central extensor tendon inserting on to the middle phalanx. Dorsal burns, rheumatoid arthritis, Dupuytren's contracture, and congenital disease are other causes.[1,2,4]

Several authors have classified different clinical stages of the boutonnière deformity. Tubiana classifies the boutonnière deformity into four stages: Stage 1, minimal deficiency of extension; stage 2, proximal contracture of the middle extensor tendon; stage 3, contracture of retinacular ligaments; and stage 4, fixed contracture of the proximal interphalangeal joint.[1]

"Littler and Eaton have explained this as a three stage process: 1) loss of the central slip results in unopposed PIP flexion by the superficialis tendon; 2) volar migration of the lateral bands secondary to transverse retinacular ligament and triangular ligament laxity; and 3) intrinsic tendon pull is now directly solely at the distal interphalangeal (DIP) joint with resultant hyperextension movement."[3]

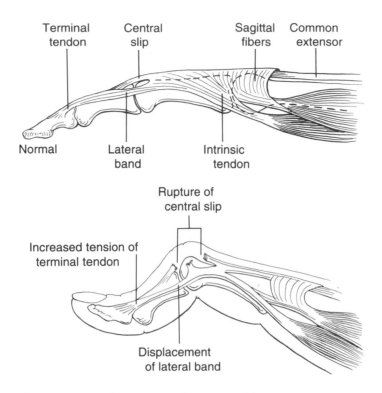

Fig. 17-1. Normal anatomy and anatomy of boutonnière deformity.

Despite different classifications and numerous surgical techniques for correction of the boutonnière deformity, it appears that most authors' treatment of choice is conservative long term hand therapy to increase PIP extension and DIP active full flexion with external splinting. Only when an acute, open injury occurs should immediate surgery be performed. The boutonnière deformity is evaluated as an acute, closed injury; an acute, open injury; or a chronic injury.

DEFINITION

Deformity of a digit in which it assumes a posture of conjoint PIP flexion and DIP hyperextension (Fig. 17-2).

SURGICAL PURPOSE

To restore extensor tendon balance where there has been a laceration or tear of the central slip near its insertion into the middle phalanx at the PIP level. Non-surgical treatment is directed towards splinting, either dynamic or static, that allows the central slip to heal yet permits DIP joint

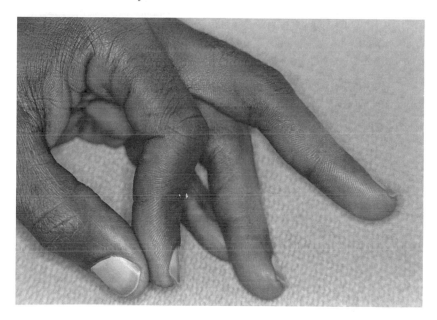

Fig. 17-2. Posture of boutonnière deformity.

motion to prevent a hyperextension contraction at that level. This form of treatment must be carefully monitored. Many surgical repairs and reconstructive methods are described. All are designed to restore the extensor mechanism around the PIP joint. Full passive mobility of the PIP and DIP joints is paramount to ensure a surgical success.

TREATMENT GOALS

    I. Prevent extensor tendon complete rupture.
   II. Reduce swelling and pain.
  III. Prevent PIP joint flexion contracture.
  IV. Prevent lateral band subluxation.
   V. Prevent oblique retinacular ligament contracture.
  VI. Restore active and passive range of motion (A/PROM) of MP, PIP, and DIP joints.
 VII. Maintain ROM of uninvolved joints of the upper extremity.
VIII. Return to previous level of function.

NON-OPERATIVE INDICATIONS/PRECAUTIONS FOR THERAPY

  I. Indications
    A. Lack of PIP joint extension
    B. Subluxing lateral bands
    C. Lack of DIP flexion—oblique retinacular tightness

II. Precautions
   A. Rheumatoid arthritis
   B. Burns
   C. Diabetes
   D. Steroid use

NONOPERATIVE THERAPY

I. Acute, closed injuries
   A. 0 to 4-to-6 weeks: PIP joint held in 0° extension with splint, and DIP and MP joints held free. Exercises as per Burton to increase PIP extension and DIP active flexion. Prevention of DIP joint hyperextension is necessary so as to keep oblique retinacular ligaments supple[2,3] (Fig. 17-3). The splint is not removed for four to six weeks and is held in 0 degree extension at the PIP joint at all times. Static dorsal splints are preferred to provide good immobilization, allows motion of adjacent joints and preserves the volar, tactile surface.[3] Volar (Fig. 17-4) or cylindrical splints can also be used. Modalities to decrease pain and decrease edema of the affected finger.
   B. 4 to 8 weeks: Gentle active ROM (AROM) exercises can begin for flexion and extension of the PIP joint. MP and DIP flexion exercises continue. Splinting the PIP joint in full extension (0 degree) must continue between exercises. Dorsal static splints are preferred to maintain PIP in position, although a wire splint (Fig. 17-5) or a dynamic extension splint (Fig. 17-6) may be worn.

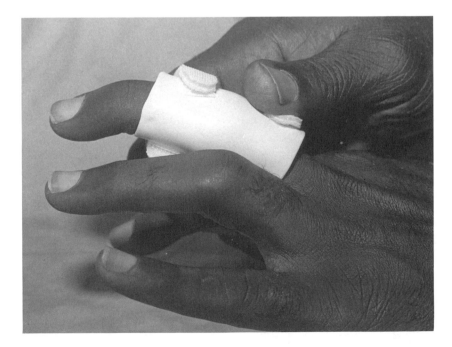

Fig. 17-3. Cylindrical splint may be worn during exercise to stretch oblique retinacular ligament.

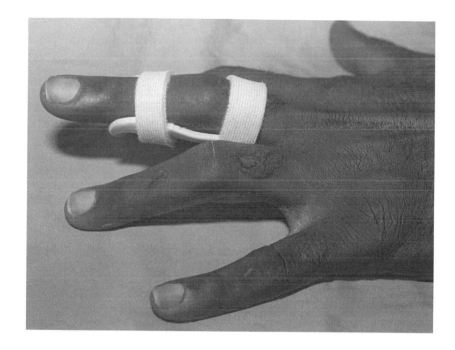

Fig. 17-4. Volar splint.

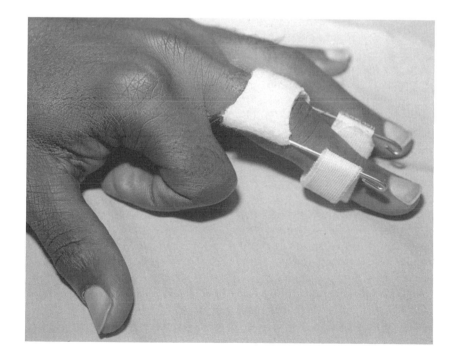

Fig. 17-5. Wire splint.

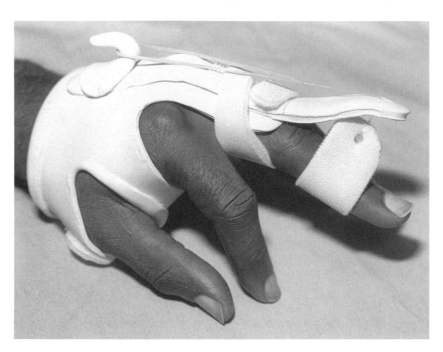

Fig. 17-6. Dynamic extension splint.

C. 8 weeks to 4-to-5 months: Continued splinting of PIP joint in 0 degree extension with active extension of PIP joint and A flexion of DIP joint exercises continuing. Active blocked DIP flexion with the PIP held in full extension should continue. 10 to 12 weeks: Gentle strengthening may begin for full fist, and blocked exercises for MP, PIP, and DIP joints.

II. Chronic deformity

All efforts to decrease pain and edema and increase ROM are attempted to avoid surgical intervention. A/PROM exercises with resisted exercise occur three to five times per day. A splinting program continues to attempt to increase PIP passive extension. Static, dorsal, serial (Fig. 17-7), or dynamic extension splints are used to attain as much motion as possible. Active DIP exercises, as described by Burton, also continue.[3]

Once full extension is attained, a static splint with the PIP joint in full extension, allowing DIP active and passive flexion, is worn to attempt to prevent surgery. This static splint is worn for 8 to 12 weeks with the patient coming out of the splint only to exercise for flexion and extension of the PIP and DIP joints. Otherwise the splint is worn at all times. If PIP contracture persists after all attempts at hand therapy, surgical intervention is indicated, first for a volar capsulectomy of the PIP joint. Reconstructive surgery for boutonnière deformity cannot occur unless the PIP joint is able to attain 30 degrees or less of extension with DIP flexion (see post-operative therapy, II)

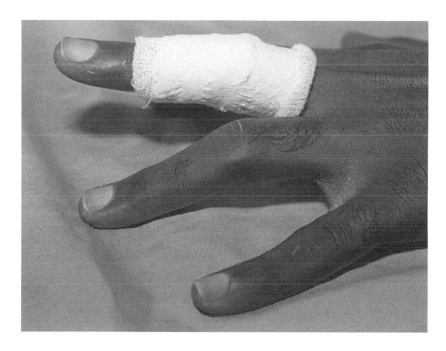

Fig. 17-7. Serial cast.

NON-OPERATIVE COMPLICATIONS

I. Deformities of PIP joint greater than 40 degrees
II. Fixed DIP hyperextension deformity

OPERATIVE INDICATIONS AND PRECAUTIONS

I. Indications
    A. Open lacerations with or without bone avulsion
    B. Failure of conservative treatment for longer than six months
II. Precautions
    A. Dirty wounds
    B. Infection
    C. Fractures
    D. Maximal pain
    E. Severe edema
    F. Previous failed surgical attempt
    G. PIP joint contracture greater than 40 degrees

POST-OPERATIVE INDICATIONS/PRECAUTIONS

I. Indications
    A. Protect PIP with Kirschner (K) pin held in extension and with external extension splint

    B. Wound care
    C. Edema reduction
    D. Restore DIP flexion

POSTOPERATIVE THERAPY

  I. Acute, open injuries
     A. 0 to 6 weeks: PIP joint is held with an oblique K-wire in 0 degree
        extension; the central tendon is repaired, and if there is skin loss,
        a local rotation or transposition flap is used.[6] Immobilization in a
        cast for 3 to 4 weeks. Cast position varies in degree by the treating
        physician but should attain a wrist extended, MP flexed, PIP ex-
        tended, and DIP flexed or relaxed extension.[1-3,6] Gentle active
        exercises begin after 1 month of splinting (with K pin and external
        splint) for PIP joint flexion and extension. The MP and DIP joints
        active exercises may begin at 3 weeks; check with your treating
        physician. The MP and DIP joints are now free, but the PIP joint
        continues to wear static or dynamic splint between exercises.
     B. 6 to 8 weeks: MP and DIP active exercises continue, followed by
        active gentle flexion and extension of the PIP joint. After 5 to 6
        weeks, PIP exercises concentrate on gradually increasing full finger
        flexion with full active extension. For PIP extension, a static or
        dynamic splint (capener or wire splint may be worn but watched
        so as not to compromise healing or increase swelling of the digit)
        is worn in between exercise sessions.
     C. 8 to 12 weeks: Active flexion and extension program continues for
        MP, PIP, and DIP joints, with gentle resisted exercises beginning
        8 to 10 weeks after surgery. If an extensor lag at the PIP joint starts
        to occur, PIP extension splinting continues. Gradual weaning of
        daytime extension splint occurs after 8 to 10 weeks, with buddy
        taping initially to allow the involved PIP joint to extend fully during
        the day. Nighttime splinting for the PIP joint can continue for 4 to
        5 months until the treatment program can be discontinued.
 II. Chronic injuries
     Depending on the stage of deformity as described by Curtis[7] and
     Burton,[2] the postoperative treatment may vary. If the patient has full
     passive extension, then only a freeing of the extensor tendon from the
     dorsal capsule is necessary. A dorsal splint for PIP extension will be
     worn at all times except when the patient gently does active assisted
     and active ROM exercises. DIP is free and continues with active flex-
     ion and extension exercises. Splinting will continue from 6 to 8 weeks
     and, if the patient is gradually weaned during the day, with night
     splinting only. If any droop of the PIP is noted, then splinting is to
     continue during the day. Occasionally, the DIP joint may droop in
     flexion; if this is noted, the DIP initially should be splinted in extension
     between exercises.

If at surgery a central tendon reconstruction is necessary to increase PIP joint extension, then a plaster cast is used with wrist in extension, MP joints in 70 degrees flexion, and PIP and DIP joints in extension. (Operation performed should be discussed with physician before initiation of exercise program.) This cast is worn for 3 to 4 weeks or is replaced with a forearm-based dynamic PIP extension splint with MP block (discuss with your physician). After 4 weeks, the PIP joint is still to be held in an extension splint, and now the MP and DIP joints can be held free. Gentle active flexion and extension exercises begin. If a droop is noted at the DIP joint, it is included in the splint in 0 degree extension when not exercising.

Splinting and exercise continue daily for 2 to 4 months and occasionally to 6 months to achieve a satisfactory result.

POSTOPERATIVE COMPLICATIONS

  I. Infection
 II. Severe edema
III. Maximal pain
IV. Rupture of the repair

EVALUATION TIMELINE

  I. Non-operative—acute
    A. 0 to 4 to 6 weeks—Initial ROM measurements are performed at 4 to 6 weeks (when physician allows PIP to begin active flexion and extension).
    B. 10 to 12 weeks—Progress ROM and strength measurements may be performed.
    C. Re-evaluate ROM and strength every 4 weeks until patient is discharged.
 II. Non-operative—chronic
    A. A/PROM and strength measurements are performed at initial evaluation. Swelling and pain should also be noted.
    B. Re-evaluation should continue every 4 weeks.
III. Post-operative—Acute
    A. 0 to 4 weeks: Initial AROM measurements can be performed when cast or dynamic PIP extension splint is removed 4 weeks after surgery.
    B. 8 to 10 weeks: A/PROM measurements can be performed.
    C. 10 to 12 weeks: A/PROM and strength measurements are performed.
IV. Postoperative—chronic
    A. Depending on the surgery performed, measurements can be performed beginning at 3 to 4 weeks for extensor tendon release from the dorsal capsule.

B. For other surgeries performed, A/PROM measurements are performed 8 weeks after surgery.

C. 10 to 12 weeks: A/PROM and strength measurements can be performed.

D. Every 4 weeks until discharge, A/PROM and strength measurements should be performed.

REFERENCES

1. Tubiana R: The boutonnière deformity. p. 106. In Tubiana R (ed): The Hand. Vol. III. WB Saunders, Philadelphia, 1988

2. Schneider LH, Hunter JM: Swan-neck deformity and boutonnière deformity. p. 2041. Burton RI: Extensor tendons—late reconstruction. p. 2100. In Green DP (ed): Operative Hand Surgery. 2nd Ed. Churchill Livingstone, New York, 1988

3. Froehlich JA, Akelmand E, Hendon JH: Extensor tendon injuries at the proximal interphalangeal joint. Hand Clin 4(1), 1988

4. Wynn Parry CB, Salter M, Millar D, Fletcher I: Rehabilitation of the Hand. Butterworth, London, 1981

5. Ferlic D: Boutonnière deformities in rheumatoid arthritis. Hand Clin 5(2):215, 1989

6. Jupiter JB (ed): Tendon injuries and tendon transfers. Section 3, p. 256. In Flynn's Hand Surgery. 4th Ed. Williams & Wilkins, Baltimore, 1991

7. Curtis RM, Reid RL, Provost JM: A staged technique for the repair of the traumatic boutonnière deformity. J Hand Surgery 8:167, 1983

SUGGESTED READINGS

Semple JC: Editorial: The Boutonnière injury. J Hand Surg 15B(4):393, 1990

Caroli A, Zanasi S, Squarzina PB et al: Operative treatment of the post-traumatic boutonnière deformity. J Hand Surg 15B(4):410, 1990

DeQuervain's Tendinitis   **18**

Bonnie Aiello

DeQuervain's tendinitis is a progressive stenosing tenosynovitis affecting the hand, wrist, and thumb. Overuse, repetitive tasks, and arthritis are the most common predisposing factors. The tendons of the abductor pollicis longus and extensor pollicis brevis are trapped beneath the first dorsal compartment of the radius (Fig. 18-1). Pain is elicited on resisted thumb abduction or extension, palpation over the first dorsal compartment, or a positive Finklestein's test (Fig. 18-2). It must be delineated from intersection syndrome in which the tendons of extensor carpi radialis

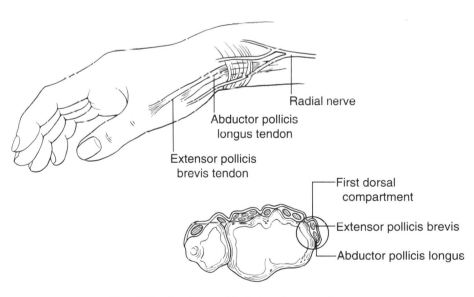

Fig. 18-1. Anatomy of first dorsal compartment.

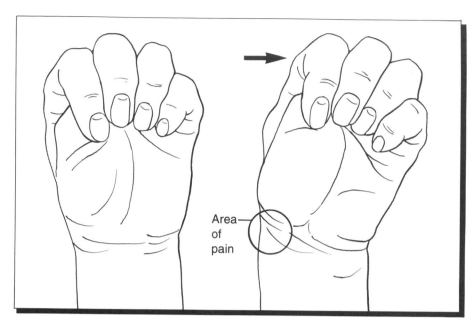

Area
of
pain

Fig. 18-2. Finklestein's test.

brevis (ECRB) and extensor carpi radialis longus (ECRL) cross under the abductor pollicis longus (APL) and extensor pollicis brevis (EPB). Pain and swelling are 4 cm proximal to the first dorsal compartment.[1]

DeQuervain's is typically an overuse tendinitis, but can be an acute injury. Conservative treatment consists of anti-inflammatory modalities and splinting, whereas operative procedures release the first dorsal compartment, taking care to release any auxiliary tendon sheaths. A change in activity may follow within the course of treatment.

DEFINITION

Stenosing tenosynovitis of the first dorsal compartment of the wrist involving the EPB and APL tendons as they pass through the osteoligamentous tunnel of the radial styloid and transverse fibers of the dorsal carpal ligament.

TREATMENT PURPOSE

To reduce the inflammation in the first exterior compartment. Nonoperative treatment is preferred with the use of splinting, reduction of demands on the thumb and wrist in combination with anti-inflammatory medications. The surgical approach releases the first exterior compartment over the radial styloid to allow more space for the underlying tendons. Occasionally an extra compartment contains the EPB tendon and must also be released, otherwise recurrent symptoms are inevitable.

TREATMENT GOALS

I. Restoration of normal, painless use of the involved hand
II. Resolution of the chronic inflammatory process
III. Prevention of recurrence

NONOPERATIVE INDICATIONS/PRECAUTIONS FOR THERAPY

I. Indications
    A. Pain or localized tenderness on the radial side of the wrist, aggravated by thumb motion[2]
    B. History of chronic overuse of the wrist and hand
    C. Positive Finklestein's test: Instruct the patient to make a fist, tuck the thumb inside of the digits and ulnarly deviate the wrist. If a sharp pain is felt over the tunnel, the test is positive.
    D. Wet leather sign: crepitus with motion of the involved tendons[2]
    E. If ganglions or triggering of the involved tendons occurs
II. Precautions
    A. Allergy to nonsteroidal anti-inflammatory drugs
    B. Contraindications to pertinent modalities

NONOPERATIVE THERAPY

I. Splinting: thumb spica (thumb immobilized in abduction, wrist in extension continually for 3 weeks) (Fig. 18-3)
II. Local steroid injections

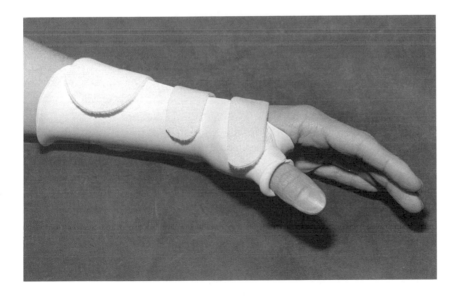

Fig. 18-3. Thumb spica splint.

III. Anti-inflammatory modalities
IV. Nonsteroidal anti-inflammatory drugs
V. Transverse friction massage
VI. Ultrasound (phonophoresis)
VII. Iontophoresis
VIII. Moist heat
IX. Ice

NONOPERATIVE COMPLICATIONS

I. Continued pain
II. Potential tendon rupture
III. Joint stiffness

POSTOPERATIVE INDICATIONS/PRECAUTIONS

I. Indications
   A. Continued pain not relived by conservative treatment
II. Precautions
   A. Diabetes
   B. Peripheral neuropathy

POSTOPERATIVE THERAPY

I. Immobilize 10 to 14 days
II. Range of motion (ROM) as tolerated
III. Scar management
IV. Resisted motion at 6 weeks

POSTOPERATIVE COMPLICATIONS

I. Neuromas or sensory deficits (superficial radial nerve)
II. Scar hypertrophy and adherence to underlying tendons
III. Volar subluxation of tendons
IV. Persistent symptoms if all tendons are not released (specifically the EPB may be in its own compartmental sheath)

EVALUATION TIMELINE

I. DeQuervain's (conservative)
   A. Active ROM (AROM) and passive ROM (PROM) evaluation at day 1
   B. Sensory evaluation at day 1 to distinguish from radial tunnel and nerve laceration

C. Pain evaluation at day 1
D. Strength measurements at time of painlessness
The above measurements are done every 2 weeks.
II. Postoperatively
A. Pain evaluation at day 1, to rule out proximal compression
B. Sensory evaluation at day 1 to distinguish from radial tunnel and nerve laceration
C. ROM evaluation at days 10 to 14
D. Scar evaluation at days 10 to 14
E. Strength measurements at time of painlessness

REFERENCES

1. Green D (ed): Operative Hand Surgery. 2nd Ed. p. 2117, 2132. Churchill Livingstone, New York, 1988
2. Alegado R, Meals R: An unusual complication following surgical treatment of DeQuervain's disease. J Hand Surg 4:185, 1979

SUGGESTED READING

Arens M: DeQuervain's release in working women: A report of failures, complications, and associated diagnoses. J Hand Surg 12A:4, 1987
Louis D: Incomplete release of the first dorsal compartment, a diagnostic test. J Hand Surg 12(1):87, 1987
Rask M: Superficial radial neuritis and DeQuervain's disease. Clin Orthop Relat Res 131:176, 1978
White GM, Weiland AJ: Symptomatic palmar tendon subluxation after surgical release for DeQuervain's Release: a case report. J Hand Surg 9A(5):104, 1984

Epicondylitis 19

Bonnie Aiello

Epicondylitis may occur at the lateral or medial epicondyle as a result of an acute or chronic injury. If tenderness occurs at the lateral epicondyle the tendinous insertion of the extensors of the hand and wrist is involved. The medial epicondyle involves the tendinous insertion of the hand and wrist flexors (Fig. 19-1).

Conservative management consists of anti-inflammatory modalities, rest, and maintenance of motion, which progresses to strengthening and re-education. Splinting may be used to relieve tension on the tendon's insertion into the bone.

Postsurgical therapy protects the insertion while increasing strength and endurance and educating the patient to prevent recurrence.

DEFINITION

Inflammation caused by single or multiple tears within the common tendon of origin. May also be the result of periostitits caused by repeated sprains. Lateral epicondylitis may be referred to as tennis elbow and medial epicondylitis as golfer's elbow.

TREATMENT PURPOSE

To reduce the painful inflammation at the origin of the extensor muscle attachments to the lateral epicondyle; or the flexor pronator origin to the medial epicondyle. The surgical approach is used when nonoperative therapy has failed. Excision of scarred tendon and removal of bone overgrowth (osteophytes) along the epicondylar ridge is achieved. Some procedures enter the radial humeral joint laterally and remove a part of the

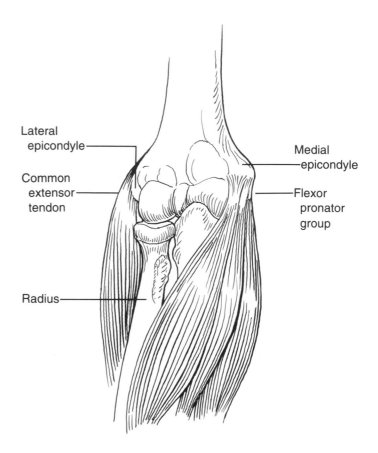

Lateral
epicondyle

Common
extensor
tendon

Medial
epicondyle

Flexor
pronator
group

Radius

Fig. 19-1. Medial epicondylitis and surrounding tendinous insertions.

annular ligament with local synovium. The goal is to reduce local pain and tenderness.

TREATMENT GOALS

I. Restoration of normal, painless use of the involved extremity
II. Resolution of chronic inflammation process
III. Restoration of strength and extensibility of the affected muscle tendon complex
IV. Prevention of recurrence

NONOPERATIVE INDICATIONS/PRECAUTIONS FOR THERAPY

I. Indications
    A. Lateral epicondylitis: pain on resisted wrist extension, passive wrist flexion, and palpation of the extensor muscle group origin. May be associated with radial tunnel symptoms.

B. Medial epicondylitis: pain on resisted wrist flexion, passive wrist extension, and palpation of the flexor muscle group origin. May be associated with cubital tunnel symptoms.

II. Precautions
   A. Allergy to nonsteroidal anti-inflammatory drugs

NONOPERATIVE THERAPY

I. Acute
   A. Ice several times a day
   B. Immobilization of wrist/hand in a cockup splint for 3 weeks (Fig. 19-2)
   C. Gentle AROM. Wrist: flexion, pronation; elbow: extension
   D. Restrict motions: grasp, pinch, fine finger motions
   E. Gentle transverse friction massage
   F. Electrical stimulation for pain control and edema

II. Chronic
   A. Restrict repetitive grasp activities and wrist flexion and extension
   B. Tennis elbow cuff: May be used on lateral epicondylitis and medial epicondylitis. (Be careful not to compress the ulnar nerve.) (Fig. 19-2).
   C. Ultrasound (may use phonophoresis).
   D. Deep transverse friction massage.
   E. Iontophoresis.
   F. Heat before and ice after activity.
   G. Stretching
      1. Lateral epicondylitis: wrist flexion, pronation; elbow extension
      2. Medial epicondylitis: wrist extension, supination; elbow flexion
   H. Education

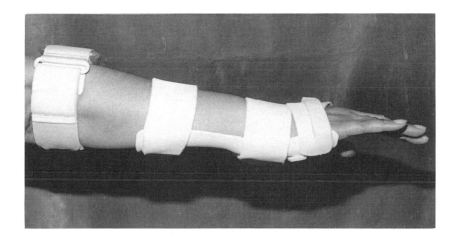

Fig. 19-2. Cockup splint with tennis elbow cuff.

III. Prevention
   A. Medial epicondylitis
      1. Increase flexor strength.
   B. Lateral epicondylitis
      1. Increase extensor strength.
   C. In both cases nonsteroidal anti-inflammatory drugs may be used with steroid injections.

NONOPERATIVE COMPLICATIONS

I. Continued pain

POSTOPERATIVE INDICATIONS FOR THERAPY

   I. Severe pain, marked and localized tenderness over the epicondyle
  II. Failure to respond to restricted activity or immobilization of the elbow and wrist (using splints, slings, etc.)
 III. Failure to respond to two injections of steroids into the epicondylar area during the period of immobilization

POSTOPERATIVE THERAPY

I. AROM in 24 hours and increase as tolerated. May return to full athletic ability after 6 to 8 weeks with tennis elbow straps.

POSTOPERATIVE COMPLICATIONS

  I. Infection
 II. Pain
III. Recurrence of symptoms

EVALUATION TIMELINE

   I. Evaluate initially
      A. AROM
      B. Pain
  II. After 3 weeks
      A. Passive range of motion (PROM)
      B. Strength
 III. Should be re-evaluated biweekly

SUGGESTED READINGS

Baumgart SH, Schwartz DR: Percutaneous release of epicondylar muscles for humeral epicondylitis. Am J Sports Med 10:233, 1982

Binder AF, Hodge G, Greenwood AM et al: Is therapeutic ultrasound effective in treating soft tissue lesions? Br Med J 290(6467):512, 1985

Binder AF, Hazelman BL: Lateral humeral epicondylitis: a study of natural history and the effect of conservative therapy. Br J Rheumatol 22:73, 1983

Boyd HB, McLeod AC Jr: Tennis elbow. J Bone Joint Surg 55-A:1183, 1973

Gaberech SG et al: Treatment of lateral epicondylitis. Br J Sports Med 94:224, 1985

Gould III J, Davis GJ: Orthopaedic and Sports Physical Therapy. CV Mosby, St. Louis, 1985

Green DP: Operative Hand Surgery. 2nd Ed. Churchill Livingstone, New York, 1988

Kessler RM, Hutley D: Management of Common Musculoskeletal Disorders. Harper & Row, Philadelphia, 1983

Kivi P et al: The etiology and conservative treatment of humeral epicondylitis. Scand J Rehabil Med 15:37, 1982

Kohn HS: Current status and treatment of tennis elbow. Wisc Med J 83:18, 1984

Nirschl RP, Pettrons FA: Tennis elbow: the treatment of lateral epicondylitis. J Bone Joint Surg 61-A:832, 1979

Shoulder Tendinitis **20**

Bonnie Aiello

Shoulder joint mechanics and stability are dependent on the muscles surrounding the joint. An acute injury or chronic misuse can cause inflammation of the tendons especially those attaching to the greater tuberosity of the humerus and beneath the acromial shelf (Fig. 20-1). Untreated, these may go on to calcify and require surgery.

Conservative management consists of anti-inflammatory modalities and rest to decrease pain and then progressive strengthening to prevent re-injury.

Postsurgical therapy allows for tendon healing, decompression of the injured tendon, and progressive strengthening and stretching to regain mechanics.

DEFINITION

A combination of mechanical stresses degenerates and causes ischemic changes in the tendon with possible subsequent calcification causing it to be prone to local inflammation.

TREATMENT PURPOSE

The purpose when dealing with biceps tendinitis is to reduce the irritation of tendon gliding in the bicipital groove of the humerus. Rotator cuff tendonitis occurs over the head of the humerus beneath the acromium process (Fig. 20-2). Inflammation caused by overuse needs to be reduced for smoother, unrestricted gliding. The surgical goals are to increase the size of this space and removal of the overlying impinging bone structures.

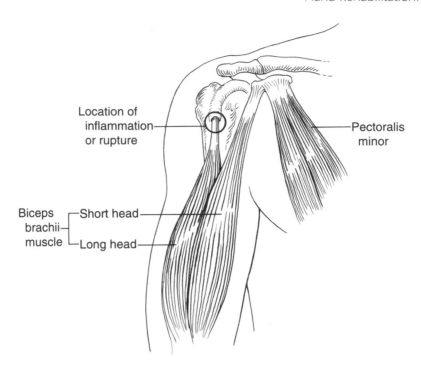

Fig. 20-1. Surrounding anatomy and location of inflammation of tendons attaching to greater tuberosity of the humerus.

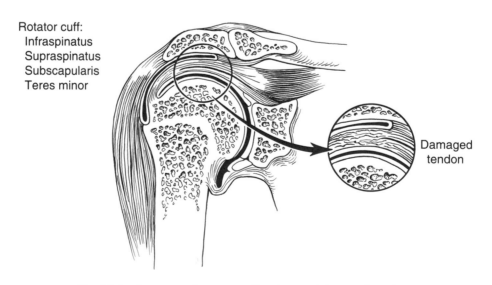

Fig. 20-2. Anatomy of rotator cuff and potential area of tendinitis.

TREATMENT GOALS

   I. Restoration of normal, painless use of involved extremity
   II. Resolution of chronic inflammatory process
   III. Increase strength and extensibility to the affected muscle–tendon complex
   IV. Prevent recurrences

NONOPERATIVE INDICATIONS/PRECAUTIONS FOR THERAPY

   I. Indications
      A. Pain on palpation of specific tendons
      B. Pain on resisted motions for specific muscle actions
   II. Precautions
      Allergy to nonsteroidal anti-inflammatory drugs

NONOPERATIVE THERAPY

   I. Acute
      A. Ice
      B. Sling (temporary
      C. Rest
      D. Aggressive anti inflammatory therapy
      E. Program of passive range of motion (PROM), especially abduction (broomstick or putty), Codman's exercise, wall walking, eccentric exercise
      F. Ice several times a day
      G. Gentle transverse friction massage
      H. Electrical stimulation for pain control and edema
   II. Chronic
      A. Heat modalities
      B. Injections
      C. Ultrasound (may use phonophoresis)
      D. Iontophoresis
      E. Deep transverse friction massage
      F. Heat before and ice after activity
      G. Stretching
      H. Education for prevention

NONOPERATIVE COMPLICATIONS

   I. Continued pain
   II. Calcifications of tendons
   III. Tendon rupture

POSTOPERATIVE INDICATIONS/PRECAUTIONS FOR THERAPY

I. Indication
  A. Failure to respond to conservative treatment
  B. Severe pain and localized tenderness
  C. Tendon calcification
II. Precautions
  A. Tendon rupture
  B. Repeated ossification
  C. Shoulder decreased mobility

POSTOPERATIVE THERAPY

Day 2: pendulum exercises 3 to 5 minutes, four times a day. Increase to wall crawling and wall pulleys. Use heat and massage as appropriate. Discharge 3 to 6 weeks.

POSTOPERATIVE COMPLICATIONS

I. Infection
II. Potential muscle tear
III. Pain

EVALUATION TIMELINE

I. Nonoperative
  A. Day 1
    1. AROM
    2. PROM
    3. Pain
  B. Week 2
    1. Strength
II. Operative (Consult physician as to surgery performed.)
  A. Week 1: AROM
  B. Week 2: PROM
  C. Week 3: strengthening

SUGGESTED READINGS

DePalma AF: Surgery of the Shoulder. JB Lippincott, Philadelphia, 1950
Gould III J, Davis GJ: Orthopaedic and Sports Physical Therapy. CV Mosby, St. Louis, 1985

Kessler RM, Herthry D: Management of Common Musculoskeletal Disorders. Harper & Row, Philadelphia, 1983

McQueen AK: Surgical relief for the painful shoulder. Aust Fam Phys 16(6):768, 1987

Rizk TE, Christopher RP, Pinalo RS et al: Adhesive capsulitis (frozen shoulder): a new approach to its management. Arch Phys Med Rehabil 64:29, 1983

Schenk's Handbook of Orthopaedic Surgery. 9th Ed. CV Mosby, St. Louis, 1987

Sinki PA: Tendonitis and bursitis of the shoulder. Post Grad Med 73(5):177, 1983

Stanish WD, Rubinovich RM, Curwin S: Ecocentric exercise in chronic tendonitis. Clin Orthop Relat Res 208:65, 1986

Thoracic Outlet Syndrome

21

Mallory S. Anthony

The thoracic outlet is the triangular channel through which the nerves and vessels of the arm leave the neck and thorax. It is bounded by the anterior scalene muscle anteriorly, the medial scalene muscle posteriorly, the clavicle superiorly, and the first rib inferiorly. The structures at risk of compression in this area are the subclavian artery, subclavian vein, and the brachial plexus. The subclavian artery arches over the first rib behind the anterior scalene muscle, and in front of the medial scalene muscle. It then passes under the subclavius muscle and clavicle, then enters the axilla beneath the pectoralis minor muscle. The subclavian vein follows the same course, except it passes anteriorly rather than posteriorly to the anterior scalene muscle. The brachial plexus follows the route of the subclavian artery, but it lies a little more posteriorly and laterally.[1]

The etiology of compression can be extrinsic (i.e., by adjacent structures), or intrinsic, from repetitive upper extremity activities and/or postures. These repetitive activities can cause perineural fibrosis of the nerves; and certain abnormal postures and shoulder and respiratory movements can aggravate symptoms by narrowing the thoracic outlet. Hence, in many cases, conservative management, including patient education (symptom reducing guidelines) and postural exercises, is beneficial. In other cases, however, surgical intervention is necessary to release or remove compressing structures.

Thoracic outlet syndrome (TOS) is difficult to diagnose because it does refer to a group of pathologic conditions, and can manifest itself with variable combinations of vascular and neurologic symptoms, frequently similar to other diagnoses. A thorough upper quarter evaluation, including status of lumbar spine, is imperative in developing a treatment program that is effective. The following protocol offers guidelines for both evaluation and treatment of this complex and challenging syndrome.

DEFINITION

Symptoms of arterial insufficiency, venous engorgement, or nerve dysfunction that can be produced by compression or stretching of the subclavian artery, subclavian vein, or portions of the brachial plexus as they pass from the neck to the axilla (Fig. 21-1).

I. Types of compression[2]

   A. Arterial: 1 percent of all cases. Two distinct age groups:

      1. Young adults, due to external compression of the subclavian artery, usually by a cervical rib.

      2. Patients over 40 in whom localized degenerative changes of the artery may result from turbulent flow caused by extrinsic pressure.

   B. Venous: 2 percent of all cases

      1. Seen throughout adulthood

      2. More prevalent in athletic males

   C. Neurologic: 97 percent of all cases

      1. More prevalent in young or middle-aged adults

      2. Females outnumber males (two or three to one)

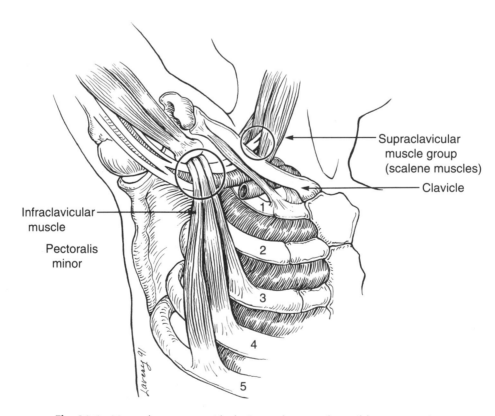

Fig. 21-1. Normal anatomy with designated areas of possible compression.

II. Causes of compression
  A. Dynamic[1]
    1. Impingement at acromioclavicular joint or humeral/scapular articulation
    2. Compression beneath the coracoid process and pectoralis minor during hyperabduction of the arm
  B. Static[1]
    1. Muscular hypertrophy or spasm (i.e., scalenus hypertrophy or spasm, omohyoid muscle hypertrophy) may reduce anatomic space for passage of neurovascular structures.
    2. Muscular atrophy: reduction in muscle mass and tone may cause sagging of local structures. (Shoulder trauma or neurologic diseases could cause muscle weakness.)
    3. Postural abnormalities: rounded shoulders and forward head are commonly seen and can contribute to neurovascular compression, and possibly exacerbate any previously asymptomatic congenital factor. Also, guarded posturing of the upper extremity can decrease the size of the thoracic outlet.
  C. Congenital[3]
    1. Cervical ribs (most common factor) cause compression by narrowing the intrascalene triangle
    2. Fascial bands behind anterior scalene or abnormal insertion of middle scalene on first rib
    3. Bifid clavicle
    4. Bony protuberance on first rib
    5. Enlargement of costal element of transverse process of seventh cervical vertebra
    6. Fibrous bands extending between cervical vertebra and first ribs
    7. Rudimentary first thoracic rib (rare condition)
    8. Scoliosis
  D. Traumatic[4]
    1. Fibrous callous formation due to fracture of clavicle or first rib
    2. Shoulder dislocation
    3. Crush injury or traction injury to upper thorax (may stretch brachial plexus and/or thrombose artery or vein)
    4. Whiplash
    5. Cumulative trauma through repetitive above-shoulder level movements
    6. Thoracoplasty surgery
  E. Arteriosclerotic
  F. Tumor in thoracic outlet: less common

TREATMENT PURPOSE

To increase the space in the thoracic outlet by postural exercises or by surgically removing bony or muscle structures that define the outlet to achieve the same purpose.

TREATMENT GOALS

I. Relieve muscle tension of shoulder girdle musculature.
II. Improve cervical and scapular alignment (restore muscle balance).
III. Modify postural habits and body mechanics that exacerbate the patient's symptoms.
IV. Return to previous level of function.
V. Prevent recurrence of symptoms.

NONOPERATIVE INDICATIONS/PRECAUTIONS FOR THERAPY

I. Indications
    When symptoms of neurovascular compression are produced and *related to arm position and use*
    Please note: The following is a list of other shoulder and neck conditions that may be confused with thoracic outlet syndrome[2,4]:
    A. Cervical disc abnormality
    B. Osteoarthritis
    C. Reflex sympathetic dystrophy
    D. Spinal cord tumors
    E. Arachnoiditis
    F. Brachial plexus injuries
    G. Multiple sclerosis
    H. Angina
    I. Blockage of subclavian artery or vein
    J. Bursitis, tendonitis, or capsulitis of the shoulder
    K. Rotator cuff injuries
    L. Acromioclavicular joint separation
    M. Median nerve compression
    N. Ulnar nerve entrapment
    O. Radial nerve entrapment
    P. Raynaud's syndrome
    Q. Pancoast's tumor of the lung
II. Precautions
    A. Infection
    B. Acute fracture
    C. Extreme discomfort
    D. Marked edema

NONOPERATIVE THERAPY

I. Pretreatment evaluation
    A. History
        1. Mechanism and site of injury (possible whiplash, traction injuries, clavicle fracture).

2. Note onset and duration of symptoms and other related injuries.
3. Detailed description of symptoms: pain versus paresthesias, etc.
4. Note habits, work conditions, and stressful conditions.
5. Note which positions aggravate the symptoms (such as overhead activities) and what relieves the symptoms.
6. Obtain results from referring physician's examination if possible.
    a. X-rays of cervical spine
    b. Pulse volume recordings
    c. Plethysmography
    d. Angiography
    e. Phleborography
    f. Nerve conduction studies (helpful if tested in both traditional resting position and position of provocation that would cause stress on lower trunk of brachial plexus)[5]
    g. Pulse palpation maneuver
    h. Social work evaluation: Minnesota Multiphasic Personality Inventory (MMPI) results and personality factors that may impact on patient's response to treatment
    i. Magnetic resonance imaging
B. Physical examination: upper quarter evaluation. Please note that mobility and status of lumbar spine may need to be evaluated because many activities and postures that are normally part of the treatment plan depend on normal lumbar motion.
    1. Visual inspection
        a. Postural assessment: rounded shoulders, uneven shoulders, forward head, head tilt, guarding posture of shoulder
        b. Atrophy: especially in hypothenar and intrinsic muscles since C_8 and T_1 nerve roots are at greatest risk of compression
        c. Color, skin condition
        d. Edema
        e. Musculoskeletal deformity
        f. Breathing pattern (i.e., diaphragmatic versus accessory muscle respiration)
    2. Strength: grip and pinch measurements
    3. Manual muscle testing
    4. Range of motion (ROM) evaluation
    5. Sensory evaluation
    6. Pain: location, type, frequency, trigger points, etc.
    7. Skin temperature
    8. Supraclavicular Tinel's
    9. Compression maneuvers used to attempt to localize vascular compression sites[1-3] (check bilaterally)
        a. *Adson's maneuver:* Clinician holds arm in extension and external shoulder rotation as the patient holds a deep

breath and rotates head toward the affected side. Repeat with head turned away from the affected side. Positive findings result in obliteration of the radial pulse and/or reproduction of symptoms, presumably due to subclavian artery compression by the scaleni.

b. *Costoclavicular maneuver:* Exaggerated military position with shoulders drawn downward and backward, used to check for compression occurring at costoclavicular space. Note obliteration of radial pulse and/or reproduction of symptoms.

c. *Hyperabduction maneuver:* Arm held by clinician in fully abducted position to test for compression at pectoralis minor insertion. Again note reproduction of symptoms and/or obliteration of radial pulse.

Note: The above three tests should be used in conjunction with all other objective testing procedures; they are extremely technician sensitive and are frequently positive in normal, asymptomatic individuals.

10. Provocative maneuvers used to assess status of brachial plexus

a. *Elevated arm stress test (East)* or Roos test (also indicative of vascular manifestation): Patient assumes the "stick-up" position (i.e., shoulders abducted and externally rotated to 90 degrees and forearms flexed to 90 degrees) and then opens and closes his hands for 3 minutes or until the symptoms are provoked.[2]

    i. *Arterial involvement:* demonstrates pallor with empty veins

    ii. *Venous involvement:* cyanosis and/or venous engorgement

    iii. *Neurologic involvement:* paresthesias and heaviness

b. *Elvey's upper extremity tension test (UETT):* tests mobility of brachial plexus and nerve roots. Clinician looks for provocation of symptoms by placing progressively increased tension in the nerve roots/peripheral nerve. Care must be taken to avoid placing excess traction on the plexus. Specific UETT technique can be found in references 4 and 5.

c. *Hunter test:* high. Tests for ulnar nerve findings (involvement of C8–T1, lower trunk). Specific technique can be found in Reference 5.

d. *Erb test:* tests for radial nerve findings (involvement of posterior cord). Specific techniques can be found in Reference 5.

e. *Hunter test:* low. Tests for median nerve findings (involvement of C6–C7, upper trunk). Specific technique can be found in Reference 5.

   f. *Medial clavicle compression:* manual compression supe-
      rior and posterior to the medial one-third of the clavicle
      may also provoke symptoms.[6,7]
      Please note that some of the provocative tests as well as
      some movements tested during ROM evaluation may not
      be tolerated by a patient with severe symptoms.

II. Treatment
   A. Conservative management
      1. Patient education to avoid symptom-producing postures and
         activities, which include occupational, recreational, and
         sleeping habits.
         The following is a guideline in reducing the aggravation of
         symptoms (unpublished protocol)[6,7]:
      a. Correct posture: patient should look in mirror, front and
         side (Fig. 21-2).
            i. Bring head and shoulder back to a relaxed position.

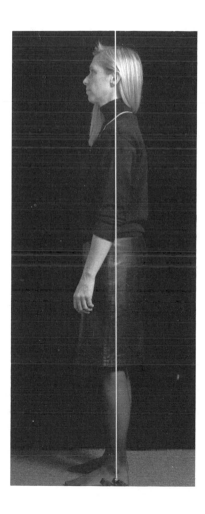

Fig. 21-2. Correct posture.

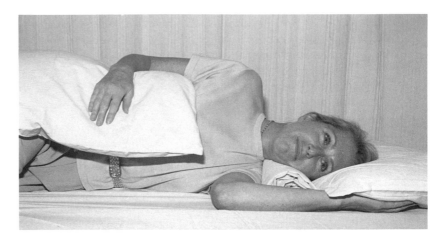

Fig. 21-3. Positioning for side-lying.

ii. Small curve in low back.
iii. Weight distributed equally on both feet.
iv. Maintain correct posture when sitting, standing, or walking (Note: ideal posture must be gradually approximated over time).
b. Sleeping
  i. Patient should avoid sleeping on affected side, in face-lying position, or with arms overhead.
  ii. A position that decreases symptoms is side lying on the unaffected side with one pillow under the head and another pillow in the line of the trunk to support the upper arm (Fig. 21-3).
  iii. Another position of comfort is lying on the back with one pillow under the head and shoulders and one pillow under each arm (Fig. 21-4).
c. Working
  i. Patient should not lean over while standing or sitting. Be as erect as possible.
  ii. When sitting at a desk or armchair, there should be a forearm-supporting surface that will not cause exces-

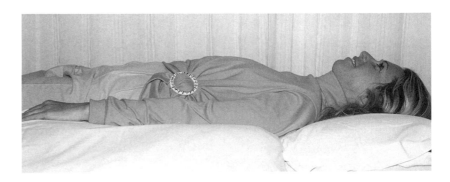

Fig. 21-4. Positioning for back-lying.

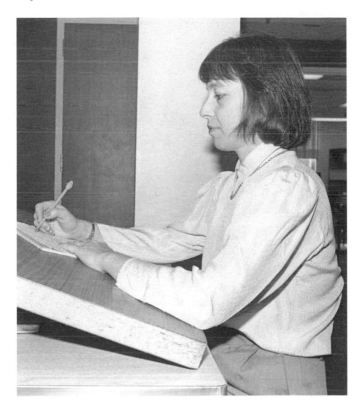

Fig. 21-5. Correct positioning for sitting at a work station.

sive elevation or depression of the shoulders (i.e., a slanted work surface) (Fig. 21-5).

iii. Patient should guard against working above shoulder level and should use a step stool to reach high objects.

iv. Patient should avoid carrying heavy objects with affected arm. Heavy items (briefcases, purses, grocery bags) should be carried with unaffected arm or held close to body in both arms.

d. Driving (Fig. 21-6)

i. Hands should be kept low and relaxed on steering wheel.

ii. A small pillow or arm rest should support affected side.

iii. If shoulder strap of seat belt crosses the clavicle on the affected side, the patient must not draw the strap too tightly.

e. General precautions

i. Stressful situations should be avoided. Stress will lead to tension of the cervical musculature.

ii. Affected arm should not hang at side while working or standing. The hand can rest in a pocket to avoid pulling down on the shoulder.

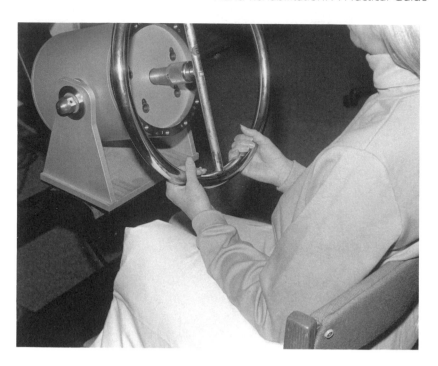

Fig. 21-6. Positioning for driving.

iii. Obesity will contribute to poor posture and continuation of symptoms.

iv. For female patients, bra straps should not be tight, and women with large breasts should have thick bra straps, strapless bras, or underwire bras.

v. Strenuous exercises that create labored breathing should be avoided, as this requires action of secondary respiratory muscles whose function is elevation of the ribs.

vi. Patient should change activities or rest when symptoms arise.

vii. Patient should have others remind him or her about correct posture.

viii. Patients should wear several layers of light clothing during cold weather. (Heavy coats may weigh down shoulders.) Cold weather creates shivering and hypertonicity of muscles, including upper cervical musculature; hence keeping warm is important.

2. Management of muscle spasm and tension in shoulder girdle and cervical musculature

   a. Moist heat

   b. Ultrasound

   c. Cold packs

   d. Massage (deep friction and relaxation)

e. Occasionally analgesics and/or muscle relaxants are prescribed by physician
Note: Cervical traction, either static or intermittent, should
be avoided as this tends to increase rather than relieve
patient's symptoms.
3. Modalities to decrease pain [e.g., transcutaneous electrical
nerve stimulation (TENS), moist heat, etc.].
Begin with pain and inflammation reducing treatments
(may need sling for a few days to help maintain rest position
of brachial plexus, that is, abduction and elevation of scapula,
and internal rotation and adduction of shoulder).[4]
4. Manual therapy to restore/increase accessory joint movement
and to increase mobility of first two ribs.
a. Joint mobilizations of sternoclavicular, acromioclavicular,
and scapulothoracic joints, as well as the first and second
rib articulations provide a reliable method of increasing
costoclavicular space.[6,8]
b. Mobilization of the occiput on the atlas will also facilitate
axial extension movement.[7]
c. Patient must be willing to make frequent visits for therapy
and must follow through with the home exercise program.
d. Techniques of joint mobilization should be performed
only by therapists with appropriate training in manual
therapy.
5. Brachial plexus gliding exercises
a. Use of the UETT as an exercise for mobilizing the brachial
plexus.
b. Specific exercise technique can be found in references 4
and 5.
6. Postural exercises[3,4,7,9]
a. Improve cervical and scapular alignment, and include exercises to stretch pectoralis minor, scaleni, and cervical
lateral flexors; and exercises to encourage scapular adduc-
tion/depression, and paracervical extension. Shoulder/
glenohumeral joint exercises and thoracic flexion/exten-
sion exercises can be added as needed.
The following is a suggested exercise program.
Exercises should be performed slowly, 10 repetitions, two
times per day to start. (If patient's tolerance is low or symptoms are aggravated, decrease number and frequency of
exercises and/or change exercise position.)
i. *Shoulder girdle motion* (to emphasize shoulder retraction): sit with shoulders relaxed; arms supported.
Make small circles with shoulder joints, gradually increasing in size. Work in both directions.
ii. *Stretching of scalene muscles*: stand erect; arms at
sides, with shoulders internally rotated. Bend the
neck, trying to touch ear to shoulder, first to right then

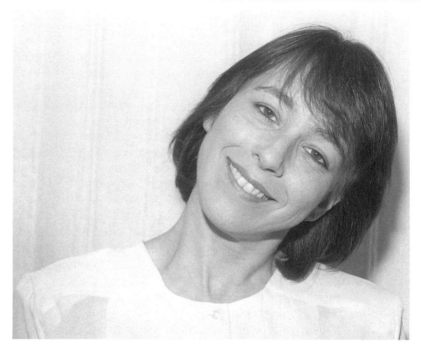

Fig. 21-7. Scalene stretch exercise.

to left. Relax and repeat. (May add shoulder depression to increase stretch.) (Fig. 21-7).

iii. *Stretching of pectoral muscles:* stand facing a corner of a room with one hand on each wall; hands at head level; palms forward; elbows bent. Do a standard push-up into corner and return to original position. Inhale as body leans forward, exhale upon return. Repeat (Fig. 21-8).

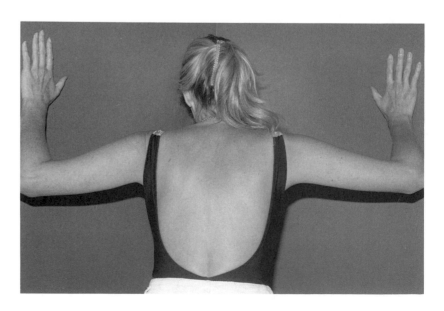

Fig. 21-8. Pectoral stretch exercise.

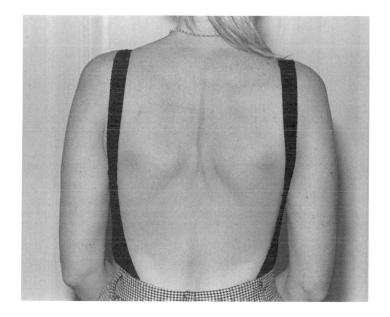

Fig. 21-9. Scapular adduction exercise.

  iv. *Stretching of pectoralis minor:* lying supine with knees bent. Keep arms level on bed surface. Slide affected arm up into abduction, attempting to reach ear.

  v. *Strengthening of scapular adductors:* sit with shoulders relaxed; arms supported in lap. Gently squeeze shoulder blades together, hold for a count of three, return to starting position and repeat (Fig. 21-9).

  vi. *Strengthening of cervical extensors:* sit with shoulders relaxed; arms supported in lap; head bent forward. Slowly extend head, hold for a count of three, return to starting position and repeat.

  vii. *Diaphragmatic breathing* (to discourage overuse of accessory muscles for respiration, which elevates rib cage resulting in decreased thoracic outlet space): backlying; one hand on stomach; one hand on chest. Inhale—hand on stomach should rise; hand on chest should stay about same height. Exhale—hand on stomach should fall; hand on chest will stay same height. Perform for three inhalation/exhalation cycles.

  viii. Progression

    A. Increase frequency of home exercise program slowly to patient tolerance.

    B. Assess progress, as often as needed (once or twice/week).

    C. Relief of symptoms should be achieved after 6 to 8 weeks of conservative management; otherwise an alternative method of treatment is indicated (possible surgery).

INDICATIONS/PRECAUTIONS FOR SURGERY

I. Indications
   A. Conservative treatment is not beneficial
   B. Patient requires narcotic medication and is unable to sleep or work
   C. Muscle atrophy
   D. Marked edema
   E. Arterial emboli or tip ulceration/gangrene
II. Precautions
   A. Malignant conditions (especially with prior irradiation)[10]
   B. Alcohol abuse
   C. Diabetes
   D. Other neurologic and vascular diseases

OPERATIVE MANAGEMENT

I. Surgical techniques
   A. Cervical rib resection
   B. Scalenectomy procedures
   C. Transaxillary approaches for fascial band release
   D. Arterial reconstructive procedures

POSTOPERATIVE THERAPY[2,10]

I. ROM exercises distal to shoulder first postoperative day to decrease stiffness and edema
II. Gentle ROM exercises to shoulder 1 to 2 weeks postoperatively
III. Mild use of shoulder 4 to 6 weeks postoperatively
IV. Full use of upper extremity 8 to 10 weeks postoperatively

POSTOPERATIVE COMPLICATIONS

I. Infection
II. Persistent painful paresthesias
III. Decreased muscle strength with atrophy
IV. Persistent numbness
V. Decreased circulation with possible ulceration of fingertips
VI. Nonunion of clavicle if clavicle is divided during surgery

EVALUATION TIMELINE

I. Initial evaluation
   A. Postural assessment
   B. Edema

C. Strength (grip and pinch measurement)
D. Manual muscle test
E. ROM evaluation
F. Sensory evaluation
G. Pain: location, type, frequency, etc.
   Repeat above evaluations every 3 weeks for progress assessment.

REFERENCES

1. Lord JW, Rosati LM: Clinical Symposia: Thoracic Outlet Syndromes. CIBA Pharmaceutical Co., Summit, NJ, 1971
2. Roos DB: Thoracic outlet syndrome. p. 91. In Machleder HI (ed): Vascular Disorders of the Upper Extremity. Futura Publishing, Mount Kisco, 1983
3. Wilgis EFS: Vascular Injuries and Diseases of the Upper Limb. Little, Brown, Boston, 1983
4. Barbis J: Therapist's management of thoracic outlet syndrome. p. 540. In Hunter JM, Schneider LH, Mackin EJ, Callahan AD (eds): Rehabilitation of the Hand: Surgery and Therapy. 3rd Ed. CV Mosby, St Louis, 1990
5. Totten PA, Hunter JM: Therapeutic techniques to enhance nerve gliding in thoracic outlet syndrome and carpal tunnel syndrome. Hand Clin 7:505, 1991
6. Smith KF: The thoracic outlet syndrome: a protocol of treatment. Am Phys Ther Assoc 1:89, 1979
7. Jaeger SH, Read R, Smullens SN, Breme P: Thoracic outlet syndrome: diagnosis and treatment. p. 378. In Hunter JM (ed): Rehabilitation of the Hand: Surgery and Therapy. 2nd Ed. CV Mosby, St. Louis, 1984
8. Jackson P: Thoracic outlet syndrome: evaluation and treatment. Clin Man Phys Ther 7:6, 1987
9. Klinefelter HF: Postural myoneuralgia. Int Angiol 3:191, 1984
10. Whitenack SH, Hunter JM, Jaeger SH, Read RL: Thoracic outlet syndrome complex: diagnosis and treatment. p. 530. In Hunter JM, Schneider LH, Mackin EJ, Callahan AD (eds): Rehabilitation of the Hand: Surgery and Therapy. 3rd Ed. CV Mosby, St Louis, 1990

SUGGESTED READINGS

Adson AW: Surgical treatment for symptoms produced by cervical ribs and the scalenus anticus muscle. Surg Gynecol Obstet 85:687, 1947
Cailliet R: Neck and Arm Pain. FA Davis, Philadelphia, 1964
Cailliet R: Soft Tissue Pain and Disability. FA Davis, Philadelphia, 1977
Carroll RE, Hurst LC: The relationship of thoracic outlet syndrome and carpal tunnel syndrome. Clin Orthop Relat Res 164:149, 1982
Hawkes CD: Neurosurgical considerations in thoracic outlet syndrome. Neurosurg Consid 207:24, 1986
Huffman JD: Electrodiagnostic techniques for and conservative treatment of thoracic outlet syndrome. Electrodiag Tech 207:21, 1986
Kaltenborn FM: Manual Therapy for the Extremity Joints. Olaf Norlis Bokhandel, Oslo, 1976

Leffert RD, Graham G: The relationship between dead arm syndrome and thoracic outlet syndrome. Clin Orthop Relat Res 223:20, 1987

Michlovitz SL: Thermal Agents in Rehabilitation. 2nd Ed. FA Davis, Philadelphia, 1990

Sessions RT: Recurrent thoracic outlet syndrome: causes and treatment. South Med J 75:1453, 1982

Tyson RR, Kaplan GF: Modern concepts of diagnosis and treatment of the thoracic outlet syndrome. Orthop Clin N Am 6:507, 1975

Urschel HC, Razzuk MA: The failed operation for thoracic outlet syndrome: the difficulty of diagnosis and management. Ann Thorac Surg 42:523, 1986

Wood VE, Frykman GK: Winging of the scapula as a complication of first rib resection: a report of six cases. Clin Orthop Relat Res 149:160, 1980

Wright IS: The neurovascular syndrome produced by hyperabduction of the arms. Am Heart J 29:1, 1945

Ulnar Nerve Compression in Cubital Tunnel

22

Bonnie Aiello

The cubital tunnel is a bony canal formed by the ulnar collateral ligament, the trochlea, the medial epicondylar groove, and is roofed by the triangular arcuate ligament. The ulnar nerve that runs through this bony tunnel is responsible for sensation in the fifth and ulnar half of the fourth digit and supplies the ulnar intrinsics, flexor digitorum profundus fourth and fifth, and flexor carpi ulnaris.[1]

Any irritation to the nerve at that level can cause severe pain, dysthesias, deformity, and dysfunction of grip and pinch strength, and fine motor coordination is affected. "Claw hand" or metacarpophalangeal (MCP) hyperextension with concurrent inability to fully extend proximal interphalangeal (PIP) and distal interphalangeal (DIP) joints in the ring and little fingers may also occur.

Conservative treatment consists of rest and anti-inflammatory modalities to decrease swelling in the closed space tunnel.

Surgically the nerve is decompressed, or moved under skin or muscle out of the compressed space. Rehabilitation is directed according to the structure disrupted.

DEFINITION

Compression of the nerve at the elbow as it passes through the area of the cubital tunnel. Causative factors include recurrent subluxation, dislocations, rheumatoid arthritis, excessive elbow valgus, bony spurs, synovial cysts, or trauma.

TREATMENT AND SURGICAL PURPOSE

To release compression of the ulnar nerve at the medial epicondyle of the elbow (Fig. 22-1). The nonoperative management is instruction in posturing the elbow, splinting, and anti-inflammatory medications. Surgical methods have a spectrum from simple ligament release, to subcutaneous or submuscular transposition of the ulnar nerve, to medial epicondylectomy. All of the above techniques are designed to remove the compressive forces from the nerve.

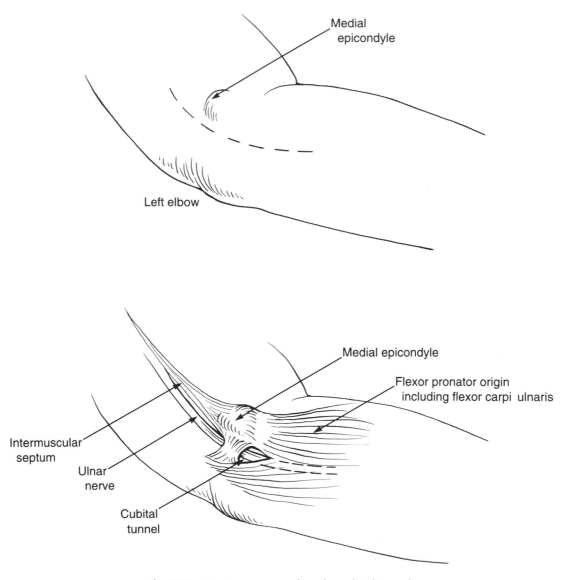

Fig. 22-1. Anatomy surrounding the cubital tunnel.

TREATMENT GOALS

I. Decrease painful paresthesias and hypersensitivity
II. Increase muscle strength to return to full use
III. Prevention of deformity
IV. Prevent reoccurrence with education
V. Maintain and educate about protective and functional sensation
VI. Increase range of motion (ROM)
VII. Scar management

INDICATIONS/PRECAUTIONS FOR TREATMENT

I. Indications
   Symptoms may be grouped into stages.
   A. Mild: intermittent paresthesias, increased vibratory perception, complaints of clumsiness or loss of coordination, positive elbow flexion test, positive Tinel's sign.
   B. Moderate: intermittent paresthesias, decreased vibratory perception, measurable grip and pinch weakness, positive Tinel's sign, positive elbow flexion test, finger crossing may be abnormal.
   C. Severe: persistent paresthesias, decreased vibratory perception, abnormal two-joint discrimination, measurable pinch and grip weakness. Muscle atrophy is present, claw deformity may be present. Positive Tinel's sign, positive elbow flexion test, finger crossing usually abnormal, electrodiagnostic testing usually positive for moderate and severe compression.
      Paresthesias radiate down the medial forearm to the ulnar one and one-half digits and compression at the elbow may be differentiated from the compression at Guyon's canal by the presence of dorsal sensory branch symptoms.
II. Precautions
   A. Diabetes
   B. Alcohol abuse associated peripheral neuropathy
   C. Other peripheral neuropathic disease
III. Nonsurgical precautions
   A. Pain due to immobilization
   B. Persistent pain, numbness, deformity

NONOPERATIVE TREATMENT (MILD DEGREE OF COMPRESSION)

The extremity is splinted with the elbow flexed 30 degrees to 45 degrees; wrist is dorsiflexed 0 degree to 20 degrees in neutral rotation for 3 months at night (Fig. 22-2). Symptomatic pain relief may be used, ROM is maintained. Splinting, education, and sensory evaluation.

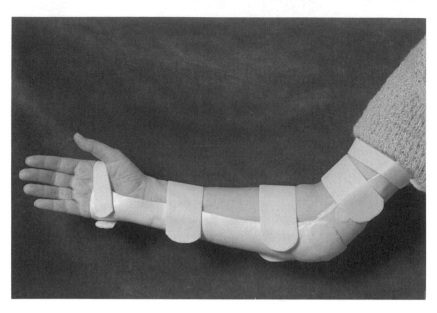

Fig. 22-2. Long arm splint.

NONOPERATIVE COMPLICATIONS

I. Pain due to immobilization
II. Persistent pain, numbness, deformity

SURGICAL TREATMENT (MODERATE TO SEVERE COMPRESSION)

I. Decompression: The aponeurosis is divided. The arm is immobilized in a bulky dressing 10 to 14 days. ROM is then progressed as indicated and is unrestricted.
II. Anterior transposition: The ulnar nerve is moved anteriorly beneath a skin flap; subcutaneous transposition or beneath the flexor muscle mass parallel to the median nerve; submuscular transposition.
  A. Subcutaneous transposition: splint elbow in 90 degrees flexion, forearm neutral rotation, and wrist in 20 degrees dorsiflexion for 2 weeks. Gentle active range of motion (AROM) is then started. Progress to resisted exercise at 4 weeks.
  B. Submuscular transposition: elbow splinted in 90 degrees flexion, forearm neutral rotation, and wrist in 20 degrees flexion times 8 days (with sling for 2 weeks). Day 9 elbow flexion only with wrist supported. Week 2 remove sling and begin gradual elbow extension exercise. Week 5 begin strengthening exercises.
III. Medial epicondylectomy: Medial epicondyle and distal part of the supracondylar ridge resected. Bulky soft dressing is applied immediately and AROM may start in 2 to 7 days. Week 2: passive range of motion (PROM). Progress to resisted ROM as tolerated.

POSTOPERATIVE THERAPY

I. Pain relief may be obtained via appropriate modalities.
II. Scar management may be started as soon as wounds are healed.
III. Splinting to prevent deformity as indicated.
IV. Sensory re-education and education about decreased sensation must be addressed.
V. Specific treatment
  A. Decompression
    1. Week 1
      a. Splint
      b. Sensory education
      c. Wound care
    2. Week 2
      ROM as tolerated
  B. Submuscular transposition
    1. Week 1
      a. Splint
      b. Sensory education
      c. Wound care
    2. Day 9
      AROM flexion of elbow with wrist supported
    3. Week 2
      AROM extension
    4. Week 4
      PROM
    5. Week 5
      Resisted ROM
  C. Subcutaneous transposition
    1. Week 1
      a. Splint
      b. Sensory education
      c. Wound care
    2. Week 2
      AROM
    3. Week 3
      PROM
    4. Week 4
      Resisted ROM
  D. Medial epicondylectomy
    1. Week 1
      a. Splint
      b. Sensory education
      c. Wound care
      d. AROM
    2. Week 2
      PROM
    3. Week 4
      Resisted ROM

POSTOPERATIVE COMPLICATIONS

    I. Laceration of the medial antebrachial cutaneous nerve
   II. Pain due to immobilization
  III. Persistent flexion contractures
  IV. Muscle rupture
   V. Infection
  VI. Persistent pain, numbness, deformity
 VII. Hypersensitive scar, heavy raised scar

EVALUATION TIMELINE

    I. Initial
      A. Pain
      B. Sensation
      C. Wound (for surgical patients)
   II. Monthly
      A. Sensory
      B. Manual muscle test (MMT)
      C. Pain
  III. Decompression
      A. 2 weeks: ROM
      B. 4 weeks: MMT, sensory, pain
  IV. Submuscular
      A. Day 9: AROM, flexion
      B. Week 2: PROM, extension
      C. Week 4: PROM
      D. Week 5: MMT
   V. Subcutaneous
      A. 2 weeks: AROM
      B. 3 weeks: PROM
      C. 4 weeks: MMT, sensory
  VI. Epicondylectomy
      A. 1 week: AROM
      B. 2 weeks: PROM
      C. 4 weeks: MMT, sensory
 VII. Repeat monthly

REFERENCE

1. Heithoff S: Medial epicondylectomy for the treatment of ulnar nerve compression at the elbow. J Hand Surg 22, 1990

SUGGESTED READINGS

Adelaar RS: The treatment of the cubital tunnel syndrome. J Hand Surg 9A:90, 1984

Baker C: Evaluation, treatment and rehabilitation involving a submuscular transposition of the ulnar nerve at the elbow. Athletic Training 23:10, 1988

Beroit BG: Neurolysis combined with the application of a silastic envelope for ulnar nerve entrapment at the elbow. Neurosurgery 20:594, 1987

Bowers WH: The distal radioulnar joint. p. 973. In Green DP (ed): Operative Hand Surgery. 2nd Ed. Churchill Livingstone, New York, 1988

Broudy AS et al: Technical problems with ulnar nerve transpostion at the elbow: findings are results of reoperation. J Hand Surg 3:85, 1978

Clark C: Cubital tunnel syndrome. JAMA 241:801, 1979

Craven P et al: Cubital tunnel syndrome treatment by medial epicondylectomy. J Bone Joint Surg 62A:986, 1980

Dellon AL: Operative technique for submuscular transposition of the ulnar nerve. Contemp Orthop 16:17, 1988

Dellon AL: Review of treatment results for ulnar nerve entrapment at the elbow. J Hand Surg 4:688, 1989

Dellon A, MacKinnon S: Surgery of the Peripheral Nerve. Theime Medical Publisher, New York, 1988

Dimond ML et al: Cubital tunnel syndrome treated by long-arm splintage, abstracted. J Hand Surg 10A:430, 1985

Eaton RG: Anterior transposition of the ulnar nerve using a non-compressing fasciodermal sling. J Bone Joint Surg 62A:820, 1980

Fanmir TF: Local decompression in the treatment of ulnar nerve entrapment at the elbow. R Coll Surg Edinburgh 123:362, 1978

Foster RJ: Factors related to the outcome of surgically managed compressive ulnar neuropathy at the elbow level. J Hand Surg 6:181, 1981

Fromisen AI: Treatment of compression neuropathy of the ulnar nerve at the elbow by epicondylectomy and neurolysis. J Hand Surg 5:391, 1980

Jones RE: Medial epicondylectomy for ulnar nerve compression syndrome at the elbow. Arch Neurol 139:174, 1979

Leffert RD: Anterior submuscular transposition of the ulnar nerve by the Learmonth technique. J Hand Surg 7:147, 1982

Ulnar Nerve Compression in Guyon's Canal

23

Bonnie Aiello

Guyon's canal is the bony canal formed by the volar carpal ligament, hook of the hamate, and the hamate. Both the ulnar nerve and artery run through this tunnel and can be affected by a space-maintaining lesion or a decrease in the actual tunnel area.

Motor and sensory deficits are present for all ulnar nerve innervated areas distal to the canal and may be distinguished from cubital tunnel deficits by the absence of any dorsal sensory branch symptoms. It may be caused by blunt trauma,[1] an occult tumorous condition[2,3] (i.e., lipoma, ganglion cyst), or a fracture of the hamate, ring, or little finger metacarpal bones.[1]

This deficit must be managed postsurgically after the space-maintaining lesion or fracture has been alleviated, with splinting, muscle strengthening, and sensory re-education.

DEFINITION

Compression of the ulnar nerve in Guyon's Canal (Fig. 23-1).

SURGICAL PURPOSE

To release pressure on the ulnar nerve as it passes from the wrist into the palm by dividing the supporting fibro-osseous ligaments or removing space-occupying lesions from the channel. Surgery also may correct fractures of the hook of the hamate or reconstruct thrombosis of the ulnar artery.

195

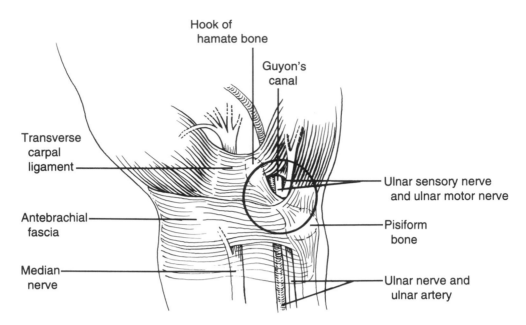

Fig. 23-1. Ulnar nerve in Guyon's canal.

TREATMENT GOALS

I. Decrease pain and reduce paresthesias
II. Return muscle strength and balance

POSTOPERATIVE INDICATIONS/PRECAUTIONS FOR THERAPY

I. Indications
    Confirmed presence of a neuropathy in the region of the wrist (especially if it is progressive); that is, the presence of combined motor and sensory neuropathy with no dorsal sensory branch symptoms.[1]
II. Precautions
    A. Nonunited fractures
    B. Malignant conditions
    C. Alcohol abuse
    D. Diabetes
    E. Other neurologic disease

POSTOPERATIVE THERAPY

I. As causes of compression of the ulnar nerve are varied, the cause must be addressed prior to the rehabilitation of the nerve injury (e.g., proper splintage or fixation for appropriate fractures or removal of any space-maintaining mass).

A. Pain relief may be obtained via appropriate modalities.
B. Scar management.
C. After protective splinting for cause of compression (times 3 days for ganglion tumor removal, 4 weeks for fracture), claw deformity may be addressed with metacarpophalangeal (MCP) block splint.
D. Sensory re-education.
E. Patient education about their decreased sensitivity must be addressed immediately.
F. Muscle strengthening may be started gradually after active range is noted and not contraindicated by fracture healing.
II. Treatment timeline
  A. Initial
    1. Pain relief
    2. Protective splinting if needed
    3. Home program of exercise and sensory rehabilitation
III. Strengthening may be started at 4 to 6 weeks for fracture or after active range of motion (AROM) is noted at ulnar innervated muscles.

POSTOPERATIVE COMPLICATIONS

I. Painful paresthesias and persistent dysthesias
II. Decreased muscle strength atrophy
III. Persistent numbness

EVALUATION TIMELINE

I. Initial
  A. Sensory
  B. Pain
  C. Range of motion (ROM)
  D. Manual muscle test (MMT)
II. Monthly
  A. MMT
  B. Sensory
III. Biweekly
   ROM

REFERENCES

1. Eversmann WW Jr: Entrapment and Compression neuropathies. p. 1452. In Green DP (ed): Operative Hand Surgery. 2nd Ed. Churchill Livingstone, New York, 1988
2. Silver M, Gelberman R, Gellman H: Carpal tunnel syndrome: associated abnormalities in ulnar nerve function and the effect of carpal tunnel release in these abnormalities. J Hand Surg 5:710, 1985

SUGGESTED READINGS

Dellon A, MacKinnon S: Surgery of the Peripheral Nerve. p. 197. Thieme Medical Publishing, New York, 1988

Rengachary S, Arjunan K: Compression of the ulnar nerve in Guyon's canal by a soft tissue giant cell tumor. Neurosurgery 8:400, 1980

Zahrawi F: Acute compression ulnar neuropathy at Guyon's canal resulting from lipoma. J Hand Surg 9A:238, 1984

Carpal Tunnel Syndrome/Release

24

Bonnie Aiello

Carpal tunnel syndrome (CTS) is one of the most frequent diagnoses seen by a hand therapist. Overuse from work, any inflammatory process, and other various peripheral neuropathies can lead to the disease. To make the patient well is the goal, but CTS is difficult to cure. The patient's lifestyle is probably the major contributing factor in the disease process. After treatment, the patient may need to alter the way he does normal activities. Therefore, education is one of the primary tools in the bag of therapeutic tricks.

Pathologic Anatomy and Staging of Compression: In early compression the epineural blood flow is impaired, causing decreased axonal transport. Morphologic changes are absent.[1] The patient will complain of intermittent symptoms, test positive only for provocative tests, and can be found to be hypersensitive to 256 cps.[2] These patients do the best with conservative therapeutic management.[2]

In moderate compression, persistent interference of intraneural microcirculation is present along with epineural and intrafascicular edema.[1] Intraneural fibrosis may be present; however, Wallerian degeneration has not taken place. There is decreased vibratory sensation, positive provocative tests, thenar weakness, and the patient complains of abnormal sensation.

In severe compression long standing epineural edema may be followed by endoneural edema and fibrosis.[1] There may be loss of fibers. Electromyography (EMG) shows denervation potentials in the median nerve supplied muscles. There are persistent sensory changes, abnormal static two-point discrimination greater than 4 mm, and thenar atrophy.[2]

These pathologic, histologic, and clinical findings will decide which path of treatment to follow.

DEFINITION

Impingement of the median nerve in the closed carpal tunnel. Usually the impingement is caused by a nonspecific flexor tenosynovitis (Fig. 24-1).

TREATMENT AND SURGICAL PURPOSE

To reduce compressive forces on the median nerve in the carpal tunnel. Nonoperative methods rely on decreasing demands on the hand and wrist to reduce inflammation of the flexor tendon synovium. This is usually accomplished by work modification, wrist splinting, and anti-inflammatory medications. Surgery is directed at enlarging the carpal tunnel by releasing the transverse carpal ligament, which allows more space for the median nerve.

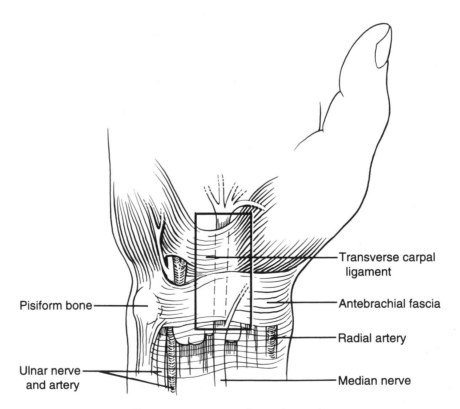

Fig. 24-1. Anatomy of carpal tunnel.

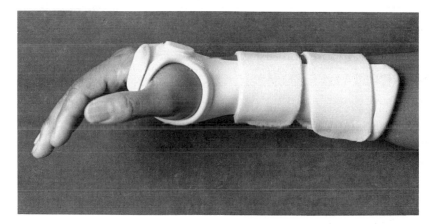

Fig. 24-2. Wrist splint for use in CTS.

TREATMENT GOALS

I. Decrease pain and paresthesias
II. Increase or maintain muscle strength
III. Maintain function of the hand
IV. Education

NONOPERATIVE INDICATIONS/PRECAUTIONS FOR THERAPY

I. Indications
    A. Intermittent paresthesias or pain, clumsiness
    B. Positive provocative tests
    C. Hypersensitive to 256 cps^2
II. Precautions
    A. Metabolic disease
    B. Alcohol abuse

NONOPERATIVE THERAPY

I. Wrist splint 3 to 4 weeks in neutral position followed by night wear for approximately the same amount of time[2-8] (Fig. 24-2)
II. Steroid injection into the carpal tunnel[1,4,6,8,9]
III. Vitamin B$_6$ therapy may be used[2,4,5]
IV. Phonophoresis[10]
V. Iontophoresis[10]

VI. Cryotherapy[10]
VII. Nonsteroidal anti-inflammatory agents[3,5,8]

NONOPERATIVE COMPLICATIONS

I. Persistent pain, paresthesias
II. Progression of thenar atrophy
III. Progression of nerve injury
IV. Decreased function

POSTOPERATIVE INDICATIONS/PRECAUTIONS FOR THERAPY

I. Indications
   A. Failed conservative treatment
   B. Moderate to severe compression[1]
II. Precautions
   A. Metabolic disease
   B. Alcohol abuse

POSTOPERATIVE THERAPY

I. Days 1 to 14
   A. Patient's wrist immobilized in neutral
   B. Active range of motion (AROM) all digits
II. Day 15
   A. Suture removal
   B. Wrist AROM
   C. Continue range of motion (ROM) to all digits
   D. Desensitization if needed
   E. Scar management started
III. Day 21
   A. Strengthening
IV. Day 28
   A. Sensory evaluation and retraining
   B. Work hardening may begin

POSTOPERATIVE COMPLICATIONS

I. Infection, dehiscence
II. Neuroma
III. Continued pain, numbness
IV. Hypersensitive scar
V. Reflex sympathetic dystrophy (RSD)

EVALUATION TIMELINE

I. Initial visit or preoperative
   A. Sensory evaluation
   B. ROM
   C. Manual muscle test (MMT)
II. For nonoperative therapy
      Repeat above tests monthly
III. Postoperative therapy
   A. First visit postoperative
      1. ROM
      2. Wound evaluation
   B. 3 weeks postoperative
      MMT
   C. 4 weeks postoperative
      1. Sensory evaluation
      2. Repeat monthly

REFERENCES

1. Gelberman R, Szabo RM, Williamson RV: Sensibility testing in peripheral nerve compression syndromes. J Bone Joint Surg 65-A(5):632, 1983
2. Dellon AL, MacKinnon SE: Surgery of the Peripheral Nerve. Theime Medical Publishers, New York, 1988
3. Calliet R: Hand Pain and Impairment. 3rd Ed. FA Davis, Philadelphia, 1982
4. Carragee E, Hentz V: Repetitive trauma and nerve compression. Orthop Clin North Am 19(1):157, 1988
5. Greenspan J: Carpal tunnel syndrome: a common but treatable cause of pain. Postgrad Med 84(7):34, 1988
6. Phalen G: Clinical evaluation of 398 hands. Clin Orthop Relat Res 83:29, 1972
7. Robbins H: Anatomical study of the median nerve in the carpal tunnel and etiologies of the carpal tunnel syndrome. J Bone Joint Surg 45 A(5):953, 1963
8. Spinner R, Bachman JW, Adadio PC: The many faces of carpal tunnel syndrome. Mayo Clin Proc 64:829, 1989
9. Green D: Operative Hand Surgery. 2nd Ed. Churchill Livingstone, New York, 1988
10. Griffin JE: Physical Agents for Physical Therapists. 2nd Ed. Charles C Thomas, Springfield, 1982

SUGGESTED READINGS

Bear-Lehman J, Bielawski T: The carpal tunnel syndrome: back to the source. Rehab Res, October, p. 13, 1988
Daniels L MA et al: Muscle Testing. 4th Ed. WB Saunders, Philadelphia, 1986
Dellon AL: Functional sensation and its re-education. Clin Plast Surg 11(1):95, 1984

DiBenedetto M, Mitz M: New criteria for sensory nerve conduction especially useful in diagnosis of carpal tunnel syndrome. Arch Phys Med Rehab 67:586, 1986

Elias JM: Treatment of carpal tunnel syndrome with vitamin B6. S Med J 80(7):882, 1987

Gelberman R, Aronson D, Weisman MH: Carpal tunnel syndrome. J Bone Joint Surg 62-A(7):1181, 1980

Gelberman R, Rydevik B, Pess G et al: Carpal tunnel syndrome: a scientific basis for clinical care. Orthop Clin North Am 19(1):115, 1988

Golding R, Selverajah K: Clinical tests for carpal tunnel syndrome: an evaluation. Br J Rheumatol 25:388, 1986

Hunter JM, Schneider LH, Mackin EJ, Callahan AD: Rehabilitation of the Hand. 3rd Ed. CV Mosby, St. Louis, 1989

Kaplan SJ, Glickel SZ, Eaton RG: Predictive factors in the nonsurgical treatment of carpal tunnel syndrome. J Hand Surg (Br) 15-B:106, 1990

Kulick MI, Gordillo G, Javidi T et al: Long-term analysis of patients having surgical treatment for carpal tunnel syndrome. J Hand Surg IIA:59, 1986

Lamb DW: The Practice of Hand Surgery. 2nd Ed. Blackwell Scientific Publications, Boston, 1989

Litchmeen HM, Triedman MH, Silver CM, Simon SD: The carpal tunnel syndrome (a clinical and electrodiagnostic study). Int Surg 50(3):269, 1968

Lucketti R et al: Assessment of sensory nerve conduction in carpal tunnel syndrome before, during, and after operating. J Hand Surg 13-B(4):386, 1988

Lundborg G, Stanstrom AK, Sollerman C et al: Digital vibrogram: a new diagnostic tool for sensory testing in compression neuropathy. J Hand Surg 11-A(5):693, 1986

Masear VR, Hayes JM, Hyde AG: An industrial cause of carpal tunnel syndrome. J Hand Surg HA:22, 1986

Mesgarzadeh M, Schenk CD, Bonakdarpour A: Carpal tunnel: MR imaging, part I: normal anatomy. Musculoskel Radiol 171(3):743, 1989

Mesgarzadeh M, Schenk CD, Bonakdarpour A et al: Carpal tunnel: MR imaging, part II: normal anatomy. Musculoskel Radiol 171(3):749, 1989

Nelson R et al: Clinical Electrotherapy. Appleton & Lange, East Norwalk, CT, 1987

Phalen G: The carpal tunnel syndrome. J Bone Joint Surg (Am) 48-A(2):211, 1966

Sunderland S: Nerve and Nerve Injuries. 2nd Ed. Churchill Livingstone, New York, 1978

Waylett-Rendall J: Sensibility evaluation and rehabilitation peripheral nerve problems. Orthop Clin North Am 19(1):43, 1988

Wild E et al: Analysis of wrist injuries in workers engaged in repetitive tasks. AAOHN J 35(8):356, 1987

Tendon Transfers for Radial Nerve Palsy

25

Arlynne Pack Brown

Injury to the radial nerve at the humerus results in limited forearm supination, absent wrist extension, metacarpophalangeal (MCP) joint extension, and thumb abduction and extension. These clinical limitations result in the functional limitation of decreased ability to open the hand to grasp.

When it is clear that the muscles are not likely to be reinnervated, tendon transfers are frequently performed. Tendon transfers transmit the muscle power of one muscle to another by moving the tendon insertion from the original muscle to that of the denervated muscle. There are multitudes of muscles available for transfer. The pronator teres muscle is usually the donor of choice to provide wrist extension and the flexor carpi ulnaris muscle is usually used for MCP joint extension. Thumb extension and abduction are commonly provided by the palmaris longus, one-half of the flexor carpi radialis, and the ring finger sublimus muscles. The following rehabilitation guidelines will be based upon using these muscles as transfers.

The result of tendon transfers can be enhanced in a number of ways. When a transfer crosses several joints, one of which is unstable, the action of the tendon transfer can be improved with an arthrodesis of that joint. The arthrodesis allows the force to be transmitted across the newly stable joint to the joints where the motion is desired. Another consideration is the phase of the original action of the donor muscle with the new desired action. It is typically easier to re-educate muscles transferred within phase. That is, a muscle that is originally a wrist flexor is best transferred to a digital extensor. Recall the tenodesis coordination between these motions during normal hand function: during wrist flexion the extrinsic digital extensors, in phase with the wrist flexors, naturally cause digital extension.

DEFINITION

Schneider defines tendon transfers as "the application of the motor power of one muscle to another weaker or paralyzed muscle by the transfer of its tendinous insertion."[1]

SURGICAL PURPOSE

Loss of extensor muscle function is most commonly associated with radial nerve interruption. It is impossible for the patient to open his hand to grasp objects with this condition; therefore, the transfer of normally functioning muscle–tendon units is frequently employed to overcome the deficit. The radial nerve supplies all of the wrist extensors and finger extensors including the thumb. Depending on the level of nerve interruption, tendon transfer planning may or may not include wrist extension. Preoperative instruction and splinting may supplement postoperative rehabilitation when the patient is knowledgeable about the function of the transferred units.

Some surgeons perform tendon transfers (internal splints) during the nerve repair recovery phase [i.e., pronator teres to extensor carpi radialis brevis (ECRB)] so that patients do not have to wait for nerve recovery to have a functional hand.

Restoration of lost muscle action by the transfer of available and effective muscle units is the goal of this form of treatment.

TREATMENT GOALS

I. Preoperative goals
   A. Maximize passive range of motion (PROM), particularly the thumb–index web space, and wrist extension.[2–4]
   B. Establish tissue equilibrium.[2,4]
   C. Educate patient about new muscle–joint relationship.
   D. Maximize power of donor muscle.[2,3,5]
   E. Maintain function and grip strength, discourage habit of using tenodesis between wrist and MCP joints for function.[4,5]
   F. Monitor sensation; if median nerve distribution sensation is absent, patient is unlikely to use transfer.[3]
II. Postoperative goals
   A. Protect transferred tendon.[2]
   B. Maintain range of motion (ROM) of uninvolved joints.[2]
   C. Maximize functional ROM of involved joints (i.e., flex wrist to 20 degrees when digits are in composite flexion).
   D. Establish firm scar at juncture site that is able to glide through adjacent structures.[3]
   E. Return to functional use of hand.

POSTOPERATIVE INDICATIONS/PRECAUTIONS FOR THERAPY

I. Indications
   Surgical tendon transfers
II. Precautions
   A. Neuroma
   B. Overestimation of donor muscle strength
   C. Less than full ROM before surgical transfer[1]

PREOPERATIVE THERAPY

I. Techniques to maximize active ROM (AROM) and PROM[1–4]
II. Techniques to maximize strengthening[2,3]
III. Techniques to maximize scar mobility[2–4]
IV. Monitor sensation[3]
V. Assess strength of and strengthen possible donor muscles[1,5]
VI. Provide splints to promote normal use of hand[6] (Fig. 25-1)

POSTOPERATIVE THERAPY

I. Weeks 0 to 3 or 4: Immobilization of elbow 90 degrees (option of surgeon), forearm pronation 30 degrees to 90 degrees, wrist dorsiflexion 30 degrees to 45 degrees, MCP joints 0 degree, proximal interphalangeal (PIP) joints free or flexed 20 degrees to 45 degrees, thumb

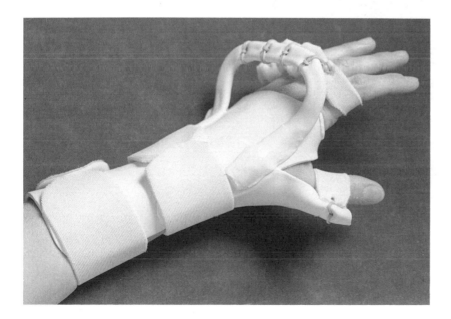

Fig. 25-1. Splints can promote normal use of hand.

full abduction and extension or slightly less than full abduction and extension (Fig. 25-2).

  A. ROM uninvolved joints of neck, shoulder, distal interphalangeal (DIP) joint

  B. Protective ROM individual joints: elbow, wrist within 10 degrees to 30 degrees of dorsal flexion arc, MCP joints, interphalangeal (IP) joints[5]

  C. Avoid composite flexion

  D. Scar management

  E. Desensitization

  II. Week 3 or 4: fabricate splint, according to surgeon's guidance, which may or may not include elbow. Position the hand and wrist in same position as that in the original cast.

  III. Weeks 5 to 6: Begin brief sessions of muscle contractions and education of transferred muscle and progress to full ROM during light pick up-release activities for digits and twisting activities for thumb (i.e., nut and bolt assembly).[4]

  IV. Week 7: Begin dynamic flexion splinting if extrinsic extensor tendon tightness is present.

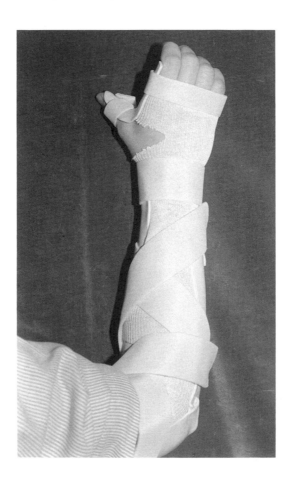

Fig. 25-2. Example of splint used for postoperative positioning.

V. Week 8: Discontinue protective daytime splinting; introduce resistive exercises.[5]
VI. Week 12: Resume unrestricted activities.

POSTOPERATIVE COMPLICATIONS

I. Scarring of tendon to surrounding structures, particularly at sites of pulleys
II. Bowstringing of transferred tendon
III. Rupture of tendon juncture[1,3]
IV. Overstretching of transferred tendon[1,2]
V. Wrist postures in slight radial deviation when flexor carpi ulnaris is used as a donor muscle

EVALUATION TIMELINE

I. Week 0
   A. ROM of uninvolved joints
   B. Protected ROM of individual involved joints
   C. Sensibility evaluation
II. Week 5: Composite AROM flexion and extension joints involved in tendon transfer
III. Week 7: Composite PROM flexion and extension joints involved in tendon transfer
IV. Week 10: manual muscle testing

REFERENCES

1. Schneider LH: Tendon transfers in the upper extremity. p. 669. In Hunter JM, Schneider LH, Mackin EJ, Callahan AD (eds): Rehabilitation of the Hand: Surgery and Therapy. CV Mosby, St. Louis, 1990
2. Reid RF: Radial nerve palsy. Hand Clin 4:179, 1988
3. Riordan RC: Principles of tendon transfers. p. 410. In Hunter JM, Schneider LH, Mackin ER (eds): Tendon Surgery in the Hand. CV Mosby, St. Louis, 1987
4. Omer GE: Tendon transfers in radial nerve paralysis. p. 425. In Hunter JM, Schneider LH, Mackin EJ (eds): Tendon Surgery in the Hand. CV Mosby, St. Louis, 1987
5. Reynolds CC: Preoperative and postoperative management of tendon transfers after radial nerve injury. p. 696. In Hunter JM, Schneider LH, Mackin EJ, Callahan AD (eds): Rehabilitation of the Hand. 3rd Ed. CV Mosby, St. Louis, 1990
6. Colditz JC: Splinting for radial nerve palsy. J Hand Ther 1:18, 1987

Replantation **26**

Lauren Valdata Eddington

Experiments on limb replantation were reported in the late 1800s but it was not until the operating microscope allowed repair of small vessels in the 1960s that microvascular surgery began. More and more reports of successful replantations occurred following improvements in instrumentation, surgical techniques, suture materials, patient selection, and in pre- and postoperative management. With the success of replantation, greater focus has now been placed on the functional recovery of the replanted digits.

Replantation is defined as "the reattachment of a body part that has been totally severed from the body without any attachments. This term differs from revascularization, which is defined as the reattachment of an incompletely amputated part, in which vessel reconstruction is necessary to assure viability . . ."[1]

After this amputation occurs, recovery of function depends on the preservation of cellular structure, as well as on the restoration of blood flow. Cellular damage may develop as an immediate result of ischemia. Extreme or irreversible ischemic tissue damage prior to replantation procedures is often seen and can be prevented by proper cooling.[1-3] Two basic methods have been described for care of the amputated part. One method involves wrapping the part in a cloth moistened with lactated Ringer's solution, then placing it in a plastic bag on ice. Another method is to immerse the part in lactated Ringer's solution in a plastic bag and place this bag on ice.[1] A compressive dressing would be placed on the stump.

When replanting, the sequence to follow for digital and hand replantation is to shorten and fix bone with repair of the periosteum (especially the volar plate if possible). Extensor tendons are repaired followed by flexor tendons. Both arteries when possible, with or without interpositional vein grafts are repaired. Finally nerves and veins are repaired (one and one-half to two veins per arterial repair attempted), and/or vein grafts, if necessary. Lastly, skin is closed without constriction.[1,4,5]

Postoperative care begins with application of the proper bulky dressing and plaster splint. A protocol of no smoking, no caffeine, hourly or more frequent color and warmth checks (to be maintained above 30°C), capillary refill, and elevation of arm to heart level with the patient in as restful an atmosphere as possible is followed. It is after the first week that the patient is referred for hand therapy and evaluation.

DEFINITION

Replantation is the reattachment of a body part that has been totally severed from the body without any attachments[1,4] (Fig. 26-1).

SURGICAL PURPOSE

Totally amputated parts of the upper limb can, under many circumstances, be reattached using current surgical techniques. Amputation causes damage to every anatomic structure. Restoration of the critical components such as bone, tendons, arteries, nerves, veins, and skin is essential for the survival of the amputated segment or segments. Not all

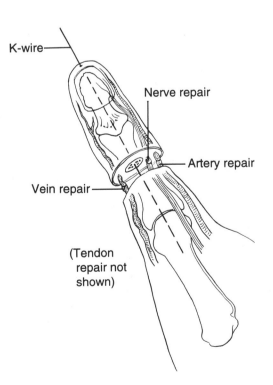

K-wire

Nerve repair

Artery repair

Vein repair

(Tendon repair not shown)

Fig. 26-1. Replantation is the reattachment of a totally severed body part.

of these segments will be suitable for replantation nor will they all survive replantation. The purpose is to restore those parts that are necessary for good arm and hand function.

TREATMENT GOALS

    I. Protect all repaired structures (i.e., vessels, nerves, tendon(s), fracture(s).
    II. Promote/monitor wound healing and care.
    III. Maintain range of motion (ROM) of all proximal uninvolved joints of the upper extremity.
    IV. Reduce edema taking into consideration vein repairs over repaired parts.
    V. Splint hand and fingers in as functional a position as is possible.
    VI. Minimize complaints of pain as indicated, of proximal joints.
    VII. Educate patient in the care of replanted part and treatment.
    VIII. Promote independence in activities of daily living (ADL) for the patient with assists as needed.
    IX. Evaluate and give support as needed by hand social work referral.

OPERATIVE INDICATIONS/PRECAUTIONS

I. Indications
    A Thumbs and any suitable digits where there have been multiple amputations are replanted, especially at zones III and IV.[1,2]
    B. All digits in children are replanted, if possible.[1,2]
    C. Individual digits are replanted where all fingers may be required for professional or social purposes (i.e., musicians).[2]
    D. Incomplete amputations of individual digits are revascularized, especially where the flexor tendon and/or digital nerves are intact.[2]
    E. Finger replantations distal to flexor digitorum superficialis insertion (zones I, II, III).[2]
    F. Limb severed at or above the wrist if (1) the amputated part is cooled promptly and appropriately, the warm ischemia time is less than 6 hours, and total ischemia time is less than 12 hours, (2) the amputated part and portion of the limb proximal to the amputation has not suffered extensive or other soft tissue injuries, or (3) there are no life-threatening conditions.[2,6,7]
II. Precautions
    A. Avulsion injuries generally are not advised except for the thumb.[2]
    B. Double level fractures, gross crush, and amputations distal to the middle of the middle phalanx.[2]
    C. Amputations in patients older than 70 years.[2]
    D. Amputations with a warm ischemia time greater than 6 hours are not replanted.[2]

E. Amputations proximal to the flexor digitorum superficialis insertion (in zones IV and V).

F. Limb contraindications to replant include (1) avulsion of the brachial plexus, (2) severe mangling injuries of the amputated part, or (3) excessive ischemia time.

IMMEDIATE POSTOPERATIVE COMPLICATIONS

I. Temperature of replant drops below 30°C (86°F), if it cannot be returned to adequate tissue perfusion, surgical re-exploration is necessary.

II. Return to the operating room within 24 to 48 hours after initial replantation, can increase the salvage rate to greater than 50 percent. After this time, the result is usually a failure and surgery may not be performed.

III. Infection: daily wound checks are done.

POSTOPERATIVE INDICATIONS/PRECAUTIONS FOR THERAPY

I. Indications

Replanted digit or part that has been cleared by the surgeon for its viability after initial postoperative dressing is removed and replaced with a lighter dressing by the surgeon.

II. Precautions

A. Change in temperature of replanted part.

B. Pressure on replanted part by straps too narrow or splint too small.

C. Increase in edema of replanted part.

D. Any changes in the circulation and/or condition of the wounds.

POSTOPERATIVE THERAPY

I. 0 to 5 days: thermoplastic splinting once referred by physician 0 to 5 days after replantation with wrist in neutral or slightly flexed position with the fingers in metacarpophalangeal (MCP) flexion and the interphalangeals (IP) in a relaxed position of extension. Dorsal splint preferred to better hold the hand in as functional a position as is indicated (Fig. 26-2). Skin and temperature checks continue hourly.

II. 5 to 7 days to 3 weeks.

A. Gentle, protected passive ROM (PROM) of wrist flexion/extension, then MCP gentle PROM protected flexion/extension and IP protected, gentle PROM flexion/extension, if there is good bony fixation. The tenodesis advantage should be utilized, that is, gentle, passive assisted flexion of wrist with simultaneous MCP and IP joint extension and then extension to neutral or to slightly

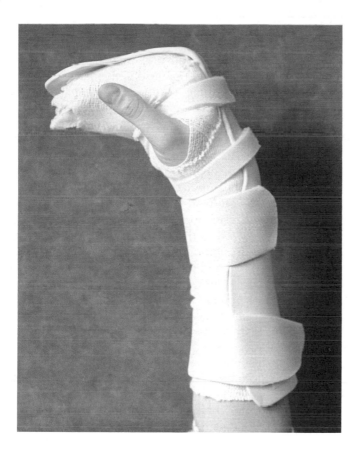

Fig. 26-2. Postoperative splint that may be utilized upon doctor referral.

flexed wrist with subsequent MCP and IP flexion. In addition, gentle, protected IP flexion with the MCPs extended (hook position) as well as IP extension with MCP flexion (tabletop or military salute), can begin passively but no active ROM (AROM) is begun until 3 weeks status postreplantation.

B. Wound care and daily dressing changes that are lighter, using petroleum impregnated fine-mesh gauze or nonadherent porous interface material and gauze[6]; no whirlpool so as not to compromise circulation.

C. Edema control by positioning of involved extremity at heart level continues; no constrictive dressings or other edema reducing techniques are begun until approximately 3 weeks or if approved by physician.

D. Skin and temperature checks continue.

E. Active, active assisted and passive range of motion to all noninvolved joints proximal to finger or wrist so as not to have joint tightness occur proximal to the replantation.

III. 3 to 6 weeks: Continuation of passive, protected range of motion for fingers and hand with active, protected range of motion begun for wrist, MCP, and IPs. Passive and active protected tenodesis exercises can continue with patient instruction in home active, protected flexion and extension exercises in the splint initially. Progression of exercises actively in splint to out of splint continues each week to 6 weeks when patient can be out of the splint at home, but should still wear the splint when sleeping or out in public. Splint may be cut down to hand based after 4 to 6 weeks if for digital replantation. Scar mobilization with fluid flushing edema techniques should continue. Patient should continue to elevate arm to heart level.

At 4 to 6 weeks patient can begin minimal gentle functional activities to pick up light objects or assist in minimal ADL. AROM continues with decreasing the protective positions and including full excursion exercise as the pre-work hardening activities increase.

IV. 6 to 12 weeks: Continue scar mobilizing techniques, as well as, active, active assisted, and passive ROM exercises. After 8 weeks, begin resistive exercises for full excursion and blocked positions. Continue protective splinting in public or when sleeping. Begin dynamic flexion/extension splinting and/or static flexion/extension splinting to increase AROM and PROM for replanted parts. Care and instruction to patient for continued circulation checks with splints on and to gradually increase wear time of the specific splints without any circulation compromise.

During this time, an initial sensory evaluation should be done as a baseline to monitor future nerve growth and regeneration. 30 cps, 256 cps, heavy moving touch, light moving touch, heavy constant touch, and light moving touch tests should be evaluated and recorded. Monofilaments are also used for further sensory evaluations. (See sensory evaluation guidelines.)

Work hardening will begin to increase use of the involved hand and gradually increase the patient's independence and work tolerance.

V. Greater than 12 weeks: Barring no bone healing problems, the patient can either simulate his actual job tasks or return to work after evaluation. All home exercises for ROM and strengthening should continue. Dynamic or static splinting will also continue as needed to further increase active flexion and/or extension. Sensory evaluations should continue every 5 to 8 weeks until indicated to begin patient on early and late phase sensory re-education. (See sensory re-education guidelines.) Discharge as appropriate.

POSTOPERATIVE COMPLICATIONS

If any changes occur as noted below, contact the patient's physician immediately.

I. Change in temperature of replanted part
II. Change in color of replanted part.
III. Replanted part begins to bleed
IV. Increase in necrotic tissue noted over repaired sites
V. Any pus discharge or any other signs of infection

VI. Any sudden increase in edema of the hand and/or replanted part

VII. Any sudden increase in pain of the hand and/or replanted part

EVALUATION TIMELINE

I. 0 to 5 days: Surgeon and nurses monitor for any changes in temperature and/or color of replanted part through observation and doppler checks. Monitor changes in edema of hand and/or replanted part(s).

II. 5 to 7 days: Protective thermoplastic splint made. Patient and therapist monitor and check temperature, color, and inability of replanted part. No PROM measurements taken at this time. Note in chart the position the fingers are held in the splint.

III. 3 to 4 weeks: Active protected range of motion measurements can be recorded. Evaluate and record wound viability, scar adhesions, and techniques used to increase mobility; also, record any painful regions and check for Tinel's sign.

IV. 4 to 6 weeks: Record AROM and PROM measurements in a protected position. Evaluate splint and adjust to increase the functional protect position for hand and replanted parts. Continue with wound evaluation, scar mobilization, and begin more vigorous edema reducing techniques, if approved by physician.

V. 7 to 9 weeks: Record active and passive gentle range of motion measurements. Evaluate joint stiffness and begin, with physician approval, dynamic flexion and/or extension splinting. Continue with edema reduction and scar mobilization techniques.

VI. 9 to 12 weeks: AROM and PROM measurements taken, early grip and pinch measurements (if bone fixation is good). Sensory evaluation and record of progressing Tinel's sign. Pre-work hardening activities continue with evaluation of patient's ability for return to work activities.

VII. 16 weeks: active and passive evaluation measurements, grip and pinch measurements. Sensory evaluation and record of progressing Tinel's (or desensitization techniques to begin if patient's hand is overtly sensitive to touch).

VIII. Greater than 20 weeks: 1 month follow-ups for ROM, active and passive, grip and pinch, and sensory evaluation with early and late phase sensory re-education beginning when appropriate.

REFERENCES

1. Urbaniak JR: Microsurgery for Major Limb Reconstruction. CV Mosby, St. Louis, 1987, pp. 2–37 and 56–66

2. Morrison WA, O'Brien BMcC, MacLeod AM: Digital replantation and revascularizations. A long term review of one hundred cases. The Hand 10(2):125, 1978

3. Smith AR, van Alphen B, Faithfull NS, Fennema M: Limb preservation in replantation surgery. Plast Reconstr Surg 75(2):227, 1985

4. Weiland AJ, Villareal-Rios A, Kleinert HE et al: Replantation of digits and hands: analysis of surgical techniques and functional results in 71 patients with 86 replantations. J Hand Surg 2(1):1, 1977

5. Kader PB: Hand Clin 2(1), 1986

6. Silverman P, Mac N, Willette GV: Early protective motion in digital revascularization and replantation. J Hand Ther 2(2):84, 1989

7. Gelberman RH, Urbaniak JR, Bright DS, Levin LS: Digital sensibility following replantation. J Hand Surg 3(4):313, 1978

SUGGESTED READINGS

Amadio PC, Lin GT, An KN: Anatomy and pathomechanics of the flexor pulley system. J Hand Ther 2(2):138, 1989

Axelrod TS, Buchler U: Severe complex injuries to the upper extremity: revascularization and replantation. J Hand Surg 16A(4)574, 1991

Browne EZ, Ribik CA: Early dynamic splinting for extensor tendon injuries. J Hand Surg 14A(1):72, 1989

Dellon AL: Sensory recovery in replanted digits and transplanted toes: A review. J Reconstr Microsurg 2(2):123, 1986

Doyle JR: Anatomy of the flexor tendon sheath and pulley system: a current review. J Hand Surg 14A(2):349, 1989

Duran RJ, Houser RG: Controlled passive motion following flexor tendon repair in zones 2 & 3. p. 105. AAOS: Symposium of tendon surgery in the hand. CV Mosby, St. Louis, 1975

Evans RB: Therapeutic management of extensor tendon injuries. Hand Clin 2(1), 1986

Evans RB, Burkhalter WE: A study of the dynamic anatomy of extensor tendons and implications for treatment. J Hand Surg 11A(5), 1986

Goldner RD, Stevanovic MV, Nunley JA, Urbaniak JR: Digital replantation at the level of the distal interphalangeal joint and distal phalanx. J Hand Surg 14A(2): 214, 1989

Jupiter JB, Pess GM, Bour CJ: Results of flexor tendon tenolysis after replantation in the hand. J Hand Surg 14A(1):35, 1989

Kleinert HE, Kutz JE, Cohen MJ: Primary repair of zone 2 flexor tendon lacerations. p. 91. AAOS: Symposium on tendon surgery in the hand. CV Mosby, St. Louis, 1975

Milford L: The Hand. 2nd Ed. CV Mosby, St. Louis, 1982

O'Brien B McC: Reconstructive microsurgery of the upper extremity. J Hand Surg 15A(2):316, 1990

Strickland JW: Biologic rationale, clinical application and results of early motion following flexor tendon repair. J Hand Ther 2(2):71, 1989

Tark KC, Kim YW, Lee YH, Lew TD: Replantation and revascularization of hands: clinical analysis and functional results of 261 cases. J Hand Surg 14A(1):17, 1989

Werntz JR, Chester SP, Breidenbach WC et al: A new dynamic splint for postoperative treatment of flexor tendon injury. J Hand Surg 14A(3):559, 1989

Whitney TM, Lineaweaver WC, Buncke HJ, Nugen K: Clinical results of bony fixation methods in digital replantation. J Hand Surg 15A(2):328, 1990

Preprosthetic Management of Upper Extremity Amputations

27

Lorie Theisen

Complete or partial loss of an upper extremity (UE) is devastating, whether the loss is due to trauma or some advanced disease. A comprehensive treatment program is necessary for the patient with a complete or partial amputation of the hand or limb. Keep in mind that each patient with an amputation has a unique set of circumstances that includes, but is not limited to, level of amputation, condition of residual limb, condition of contralateral limb, and stage of adjustment to the loss.

DEFINITION

The initial phase of rehabilitation begins during the initial hospitalization. Later phases of rehabilitation usually occur in an outpatient setting. As a result of the typically shorter inpatient stay, many initial phase treatment goals will be addressed as an outpatient.

SURGICAL PURPOSE

To remove useless or nonviable extremity parts that have been severely damaged by disease or trauma. Amputations are commonly performed for life-threatening infections, irreversible vascular compromise, tissue damage beyond hope of repair, and advanced loss of function so that the extremity becomes a biologic parasite for the patient (Fig. 27-1). Rarely chronic pain is a reason for amputation. The level of amputation is important and must be determined by the surgeon. The more length that can be safely preserved, the better the prognosis for efficient and compliant prosthetic wear and use.

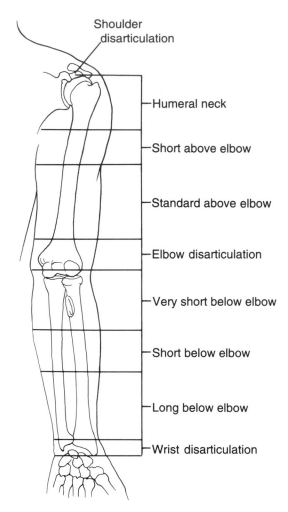

Fig. 27-1. Upper extremity amputations are performed for useless or nonviable parts severely damaged by disease or trauma.

TREATMENT PURPOSE

  I. Promote early mobilization
  II. Promote proper shaping of the residual stump
  III. Maximize independence in activities of daily living (ADL)
  IV. Provide orientation to the next rehabilitation phase (i.e., initial phase rehabilitation should orient the patient to follow up with outpatient treatment)
  V. Introduce options regarding UE prosthesis, if indicated

TREATMENT GOALS

  I. Promote wound healing
 II. Reduce edema of residual stump
III. Control or reduce incisional and phantom pain
IV. Maintain or increase active range of motion (AROM) and passive range of motion (PROM)
 V. Promote ADL independence
VI. Explore patient's and family's feelings regarding loss of limb
VII. Explore resources for continuation of preprosthetic training, prosthetic training, and other necessary services

POSTOPERATIVE INDICATIONS/PRECAUTIONS FOR THERAPY

 I. Indications
    A. Any patient with an amputation, complete or partial, who is otherwise medically stable and able to participate in ADL and exercise programs
II. Precautions
    A. Unstable medical status
    B. Others as noted by physician

POSTOPERATIVE THERAPY

I. Evaluation
    A. Data base should include age, sex, hand dominance, occupation, avocations, date of injury, date of surgery, level of amputation, mechanism of injury, current medical status, past medical history.
    B. Note skin condition at site of amputation. Note other structures (i.e., tendon or bone) that may have suffered trauma in both upper extremities.
    C. Presence of edema, girth measurements.
    D. Range of motion (ROM) of residual joints and of sound UE. Pay special attention to shoulder girdle and radioulnar joints, particularly if amputation is proximal to or at the wrist.
    E. Muscle strength of residual musculature and of sound UE. Adhere to precautions with respect to orthopedic condition and other soft tissue injuries.
    F. Presence and quality or description of pain.
    G. Sensibility and hypersensitivity at stump.
    H. ADL status.
    I. Posture and balance.
    J. Note the need for additional support from a social worker or psychologist.

  II. Treatment plan
    A. Wound care as prescribed by physician. Adhere to special precautions (e.g., skin graft).
    B. Edema control: consider use of compression pump, elevation, and stump wrapping as condition of vascular system and soft tissues allows.
    C. Splinting as necessary for protecting any repaired structures or for decreasing limitations in ROM.
    D. Active, active assistive, or passive range of motion exercise program as indicated, paying special attention to shoulder girdle and radio–ulnar joints.
    E. Consider transcutaneous electric nerve stimulator (TENS) for pain control.
    F. Desensitization program as condition of wounds allows.
    G. ADL training should include compensatory techniques and adaptive equipment. Consider use of temporary pylon to aid in ADL independence.
    H. Postural exercises, if indicated.
    I. Initiate appropriate intervention from a social worker, psychologist, or psychiatrist.
 III. Discharge planning evaluation from inpatient unit
    A. Identify initial problems and any additional problems.
    B. Note progress or lack of progress; include explanation for lack of progress (e.g., complications).
    C. Potential for additional rehabilitation.
    D. Follow-up plan.
      1. Location and date of initial visit for further outpatient rehabilitation
      2. Follow-up with primary surgeon
      3. Social work, psychologist, or psychiatrist follow-up as indicated
      4. Appointment for amputee clinic or physiatrist appointment for prosthetic prescription and other necessary services

POSTOPERATIVE COMPLICATIONS

  I. Infection
 II. Delayed healing
III. Decreased ROM due to immobilization period
IV. Neuroma and other scar adherence problems

EVALUATION TIMELINE

  I. Initial assessment when medically stable.
 II. Re-evaluation every week thereafter during initial phase of rehabilitation.
III. In late phases or rehabilitation, re-evaluate at least monthly.

SUGGESTED READINGS

Atkins D, Meir III R: Comprehensive Management of the Upper Extremity Amputee. Springer-Verlag, New York, 1989

Helpa M: The Union Memorial Hospital Lower Extremity Amputee Program, Baltimore, 1990

Olivett B: Adult amputee management and conventional prosthetic training. p. 1057. In Hunter J, Schneider L, Mackin E: Rehabilitation of the Hand: Surgery and Therapy, 3rd Ed. CV Mosby, St. Louis, 1990

Upper Limb Prosthetics. 2nd Revision. New York University Post-Graduate Medical School, New York, 1986

Partial Digit Amputation 28

Linda Coll Ware

Partial digit amputations are the most common type of amputation seen in the upper extremity.[1] There are various ways to treat these injuries, such as: split-thickness skin grafts, bone shortening with primary closure, healing by secondary intention, V–Y flap, volar flap, cross-finger flap, thenar flap, and hypothenar flap.[1–4] Regardless of surgical technique, the goals of surgery are (1) preservation of functional length, (2) preservation of useful sensibility, (3) prevention of symptomatic neuromas, (4) prevention of adjacent joint contractures, (5) short morbidity, (6) early return of the patient to work or play.[1]

Partial digit amputations can occur at different levels. The level of the amputation can affect the amount of recoverable movement. If the amputation is distal to the sublimis insertion, the middle phalanx segment will be able to participate effectively in grasping activities. However, if the amputation occurs proximal to the insertion, there will be no active flexion of the remaining middle phalanx. Once an amputation has occurred proximal to the proximal interphalangeal (PIP) joint the remaining proximal segment is controlled by the intrinsic muscles and the extensor digitorum communis. This may only allow 45 degrees of active flexion of the metacarpophalangeal (MCP) joint. If the amputation occurs at the MCP level, the patient is left with a space that make it difficult to keep small objects in the palm. At this point a ray resection may be considered.[1]

Loss of a digit can be devastating for the patient. Emotional support and a referral to social work or psychiatry may be necessary.

DEFINITION

Partial digit amputation is the loss of skin or pulp, or with exposed bone of the finger (Fig. 28-1).

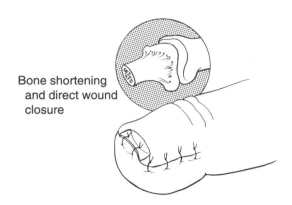

Bone shortening
and direct wound
closure

Fig. 28-1. Digital amputation.

SURGICAL PURPOSE

Badly damaged fingers may require partial amputations to remove devitalized or infected tissues that are irreparable or irretrievable. In cases of sharp digital injuries, when replantation is not possible, an amputation with soft tissue closure is required. Closure of amputation stumps may require soft tissue advancement flaps, skin grafts, or skeletal shortening. Trimming and protection of nerve ends is frequently required. It is very important to maintain the integrity and mobility of the more proximal joints for optimum hand function.

TREATMENT GOALS

   I. Promote wound closure and optimal scar formation
  II. Maintain full range of motion (ROM) of all uninvolved joints
 III. Maximize ROM of all involved joints
 IV. Desensitization/sensory re-education of injured tip
  V. Return patient to previous level of function

NONOPERATIVE INDICATIONS/PRECAUTIONS FOR THERAPY

  I. Indications
      Partial digit amputations allowed to heal by secondary intention
 II. Precautions
    A. Exposed bone
    B. Associated nail bed injury
    C. Associated fractures
    D. Associated nerve lacerations
    E. Associated tendon lacerations

NONOPERATIVE THERAPY

I. Wound care (see Ch. 1)
II. Protective splinting
III. ROM
IV. Edema control
V. Desensitization/sensory re-education
VI. Scar management once wound is healed
VII. Strengthening
VIII. Fine motor and functional activities

NONOPERATIVE COMPLICATIONS

I. Infection
II. Prolonged open wound
III. Hypersensitivity
IV. Diminished sensation
V. Neuroma
VI. Poorly shaped tip
VII. Adherent scar
VIII. Limited ROM
IX. Alienation of digit

POSTOPERATIVE INDICATIONS/PRECAUTIONS FOR THERAPY

I. Indications
   Partial digit amputations closed by sutures, skin grafts, or flaps
II. Precautions
   A. Presence of graft or flap
   B. Associated nail bed injuries
   C. Associated fractures
   D. Associated nerve lacerations
   E. Associated tendon lacerations

POSTOPERATIVE THERAPY

I. Wound care including donor site
II. Protective splinting
III. Edema control
IV. ROM
V. Desensitization/sensory re-education
VI. Scar management once wound is closed
VII. Strengthening
VIII. Fine motor and functional activities

POSTOPERATIVE COMPLICATIONS

   I. Graft or flap infection, hematoma, necrosis
  II. Donor site infection
 III. Hypersensitivity in fingertip and/or donor site
 IV. Diminished sensation in fingertip and/or donor site
  V. Neuroma
 VI. Poorly shaped tip
VII. Adherent scar
VIII. Limited ROM
 IX. Alienation of digit

EVALUATION TIMELINE

  I. Nonoperative
    A. Immediately
      1. Wound assessment
      2. Active ROM (AROM) and passive ROM (PROM) measurements of all joints
    B. Once wound is healed
      1. Scar assessment
      2. AROM and PROM measurements of all joints
      3. Strength measurements
      4. Sensory evaluation
      5. Fine motor and functional assessments
 II. Operative
    A. Immediately
      1. Wound assessment including donor site.
      2. AROM and PROM of uninvolved joints.
      * ROM of involved joints may be delayed until graft or flap is well established. Consult physician.
    B. Once graft or flap is well established
      1. Scar assessment
      2. AROM and PROM of all joints
      3. Stength measurements
      4. Sensory evaluation
      5. Fine motor and functional assessments

REFERENCES

1. Louis DS: Amputations. p. 55. In Green DP (ed): Operative Hand Surgery. Churchill Livingstone, New York, 1982
2. Beasley RW: Surgery of hand and finger amputations. Orthop Clin North Am 12(4):763, 1981
3. Schenck RR, Cheema TA: Hypothenar skin grafts for fingertip reconstruction. J Hand Surg 9A:750, 1984
4. Tupper J, Miller G: Sensitivity following volar V-Y plasty for fingertip amputations. J Hand Surg 10-B:183, 1985

Total Shoulder Arthroplasty 29

Anne Edmonds

Total shoulder arthroplasty is a procedure that is used to provide a painless range of motion (ROM) by replacing the humeral head and glenoid articulating surface. The population that receives this arthroplasty is that with rheumatoid arthritis, severely comminuted fractures of the humeral head, osteoarthritis, avascular necrosis, sickle cell infarction, irradiation necrosis, ochronosis, and gout (Fig. 29-1).

DEFINITION

Replacement of the humeral head and the glenoid articulating surface with prosthetic components.

Three types of replacement components

I. Unconstrained: used with polyethylene glenoid component that conforms to the radius of the glenoid articulating surface. Unconstrained components have replaced semiconstrained and constrained due to the problem of loosening of the latter two (Figs. 29-2 and 29-3). This is the most extensively used component.
II. Semiconstrained: monospherical. The humeral head is smaller and spherical with a head neck angle of 60 degrees and reportedly permits increased ROM. The glenoid component is matched to the humeral head prosthesis to allow constant surface contact.[1]
III. Constrained: designed for patients who have severe deterioration without a reconstructible rotator cuff but with a functioning deltoid muscle.

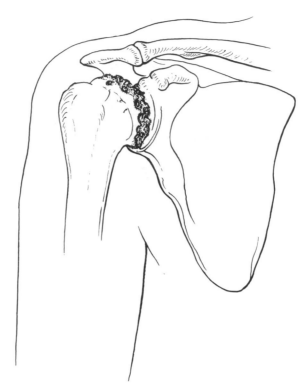

Fig. 29-1. Arthritis of a gleno-humeral joint of shoulder.

Arthritic shoulder joint

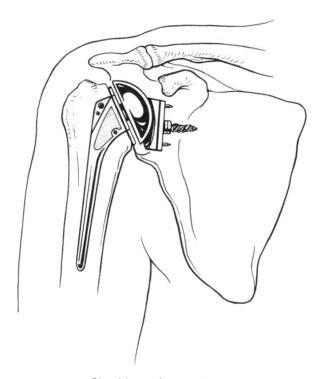

Fig. 29-2. Unconstrained prosthesis of shoulder.

Shoulder replacement

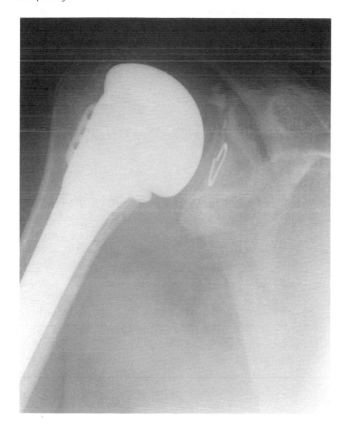

Fig. 29-3. X-ray of unconstrained shoulder prosthesis.

SURGICAL PURPOSE

To remove painful irregular and deformed gleno-humeral joint surfaces and replace them with metal or plastic. Restoration approximating normal skeletal alignment and joint stability with an effective, pain-free ROM is derived.

TREATMENT GOALS

I. To concentrate on the rehabilitation of the soft tissues encompassing the implant and emphasize the importance of the reconstruction
II. To restore pain-free ROM
III. To increase function

POSTOPERATIVE INDICATIONS/PRECAUTIONS FOR THERAPY

I. Indications
   A. Decreased ROM and function

II. Precautions
   A. Infection
   B. Integrity of muscle tissue surrounding the implant
   C. Stability of implant

POSTOPERATIVE THERAPY: UNCONSTRAINED PROSTHESIS

I. Phase I
   A. Local heat and passive or assisted motion exercises begun days 1 to 6.
   B. Exercise in external rotation to neutral and flexion initiated on fourth or fifth day with the patient supine. External rotation should not go beyond neutral for first 3 weeks. Motion is assisted by opposite hand and later a cane.
   C. At 7 days, pendulum exercises are added: with the body in a forward flexed position, circles are made with the upper extremity in external rotation and then internal rotation.
II. Phase II
   A. At 8 to 10 days, initiation of exercise performed in standing position. Hyperextension exercise is begun, assisted by both hands overhead. Pulley exercise is initiated for shoulder flexion. Internal rotation begun also.
   B. At 14 to 16 days, horizontal external rotation is begun with the patient in supine position.
   C. At 17 to 21 days, begin isometric exercises with elbows flexed to 90 degrees and held close to the body. The opposite hand, wall, or door jamb can provide resistance.
III. Phase III
   A. At 6 weeks, gradual active exercise for deltoid and subscapularis is begun. Attempt flexion in sitting position if it can easily be performed in supine.
   B. Mild resistance may be added progressing from active to resistive exercise.
   C. With gradual increase in strength, increase stretching and strengthening exercises.
   D. To achieve maximum function, 12 to 18 months of vigorous regular exercise is required.

POSTOPERATIVE COMPLICATIONS

I. Infection
II. Excessive paralysis with complete loss of function of both the deltoid and the rotator cuff[2]

EVALUATION TIMELINE

I. Phase I
   A. 1 to 6 days: passive assisted motion exercises in flexion. No external rotation or abduction past 90 degrees.
   B. 4 to 5 days: assisted external rotation and flexion exercises initiated in supine position. No external rotation beyond neutral for first 3 weeks.
   C. 7 days: pendulum exercises.
II. Phase II
   A. 8 to 10 days: exercises in standing position. Hyperextension exercise assisted by both hands using a cane. Overhead pulley exercise initiated.
   B. 14 to 16 days: horizontal external rotation with patient supine.
   C. 17 to 21 days: isometric exercise with elbows flexed to 90 degrees and held close to body. Resistance may be given by opposite hand, wall, or door jamb.
III. Phase III
   A. 6 weeks: gradual active exercise for deltoid and subscapularis; flexion exercise in sitting position if easily performed in supine; mild resistance may be added.
   B. 12 to 18 months: total vigorous regular exercise to achieve maximum motion.

REFERENCES

1. Clayton ML, Ferlie DC, Jeffers PD: Prosthetic arthroplasties of the shoulder. Clin Orthop Relat Res 164:184, 1982
2. Sisk TD, Wright PE: Arthroplasty of shoulder and elbow. p. 1503. In: Campbells Operative Orthopedics. Vol. II. CV Mosby, St Louis, 1987

SUGGESTED READINGS

Neer CS, Kirby RM: Revision of humeral head and total shoulder arthroplasties. Clin Orthop Relat Res 170:189, 1982
Neer CS, Watson KC, Stanton FJ: Recent experience in total shoulder replacement. J Bone Joint Surg 64-a(3):319, 1982

Total Elbow Arthroplasty 30

Anne Edmonds

Since 1974, total elbow arthroplasties have been performed on post-traumatic, osteoarthritis, and rheumatoid patients (Fig. 30-1). The primary goal is to obtain an effective range of motion (ROM) with diminished pain.

DEFINITION

Prosthesis that attempts, to varying degrees, to duplicate the designer's concept of the important features of surface anatomy.

Prostheses can be divided into three basic types:

I. Constrained: Constructed with either metal-to-metal or metal-to-high density polyethylene, through a bushing or a separate polyethylene piece.[1] This type of prosthesis is rarely used.
II. Semi-constrained: Also a hinge, but allows a few degrees lateral motion. This type was designed to help alleviate some of the loosening problems found with constrained hinges[1] (Figs. 30-2 to 30-4).
III. Unconstrained: Consists of separate units of metal-to-high density polyethylene components. Some are designed to be used with a radial head replacement[1] (Figs. 30-5 and 30-6).

SURGICIAL PURPOSE

To remove the irregular and painful ulna–humeral joint and replace these surfaces with new, usually metal or plastic, surfaces. The radial head is excised and often not replaced to improve pronation and supination. Joint stability is restored and a painless but effective ROM is derived.

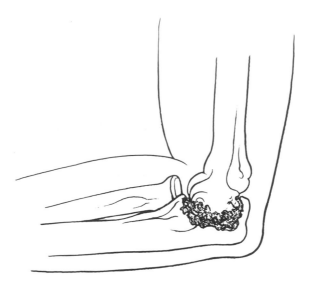

Fig. 30-1. Arthritis of elbow joint.

Semi-
constrained

Fig. 30-2. Semiconstrained elbow
prosthesis.

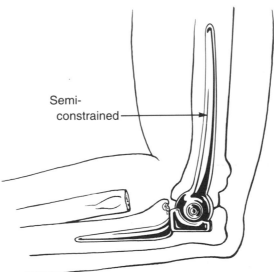

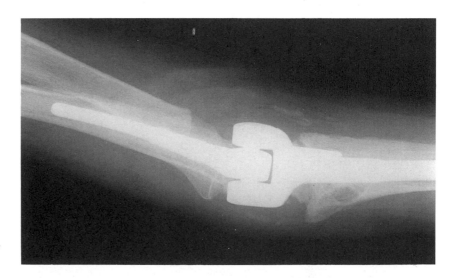

Fig. 30-3. Anterior/posterior X-ray
of semi-constrained prosthesis.

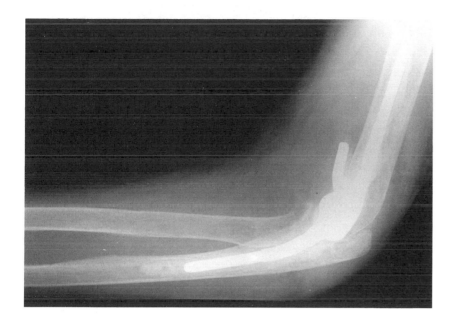

Fig. 30-4. Lateral X-ray of same semi-constrained prosthesis.

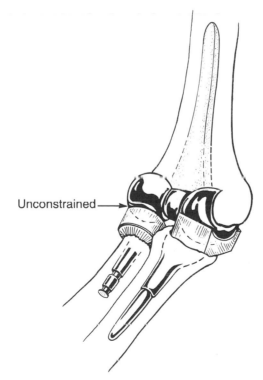

Unconstrained

Fig. 30-5. Unconstrained elbow prosthesis.

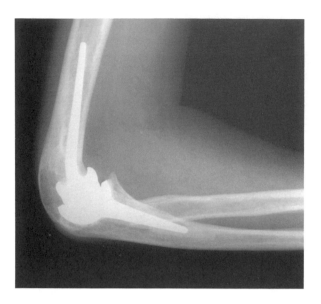

Fig. 30-6. X-ray of unconstrained capito–condylar elbow prosthesis.

TREATMENT GOALS

I. Regain maximum elbow ROM to within the limits of the prosthesis
II. Regain maximum strength
III. Enable the patient to become proficient in self-care skills
IV. Assess the patient's home environment for proper discharge

POSTOPERATIVE INDICATIONS/PRECAUTIONS FOR THERAPY

I. Indications
   A. Immobilization of nonconstrained arthroplasty for 2 to 3 weeks may be necessary if instability is a problem. Usually protected motion is initiated at 3 to 5 days if ligament repair is stable.
   B. Mobilization begins earlier in a rheumatoid patient with history of stiff joints versus lax joints.
   C. If ligaments were detached and reattached the elbow is protected for 6 weeks.
   D. Elbow motion in the rheumatoid patient is generally better following arthroplasty than a patient with traumatic open reduction internal fixation.[1]
II. Precautions
   A. Stability of ligamentous repair
   B. Clinical manifestations and selected surgical repair
   C. Avoidance of angular stress or torque on elbow when moving
   D. Regain maximum elbow flexion while eliminating stress on triceps repair

POSTOPERATIVE THERAPY

I. Nonconstrained elbow prosthesis has had problem with instability and therefore immobilization is usually 2 to 3 weeks. If ligaments were detached and reattached, protection for 6 weeks.

II. Splint applied in a comfortable position immediately postoperatively depending on procedure used; for example, if triceps were taken down then elbow is positioned in 0 degree; if Kolker procedure used, then splint position will be about 70 degrees.

III. Immediate active ROM (AROM) to hand and wrist only.

IV. At 3 to 5 days: begin protected active assisted elbow flexion/extension if ligamentous repair is stable.

V. At 5 to 8 days: begin gentle passive extension and active assisted supination/pronation.

VI. At 5 to 8 days: begin simple activities of daily living (ADL), keep arm adducted, can move shoulder slightly. Use sling up to 6 weeks.

VII. At 12 to 14 days: eat with fingers, buttoning, some grooming.

VIII. At 14 to 15 days: if little or no pain, begin graded resistive exercise for fingers.

IX. At three and one-half to 4 weeks: keep arm adducted while performing exercise. May discontinue day splint at 4 weeks, continue at night to 6 weeks.

X. At 5 to 6 weeks: begin resistive activities in pure planar exercise motions, isometrics at 6 to 7 weeks.

XI. 6 to 8 weeks: begin continuous passive motion (CPM) (Fig. 30-7).

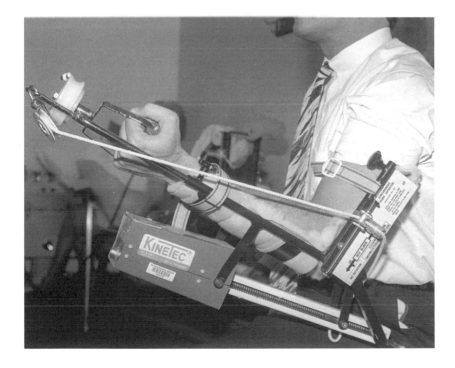

Fig. 30-7. CPM may be used in postoperative treatment.

XII. Up to 6 months: no lifting, jarring, pounding, pushing, or weight bearing.
XIII. Restrictions
    A. No racquet sports
    B. No golf or bowling
    C. No competitive sport activities
    D. No heavy labor

POSTOPERATIVE COMPLICATIONS

I. Infection
II. Triceps weakness
III. Ulnar neuropathy
IV. Prosthesis loosening

EVALUATION TIMELINE

I. Active ROM of hand and wrist can be measured immediately.
II. Immediate AROM to hand and wrist only.
III. Active assisted ROM of elbow can be measured at 3 to 5 days.
IV. 5 to 8 days: Begin gentle passive extension and active assisted supination/pronation. Passive extension can be measured. ROM should be measured thereafter every 2 weeks.
V. 14 to 15 days: Begin graded resistive exercises to fingers.
VI. 5 to 6 weeks: resistive exercises in pure planar exercise motions.
VII. 6 to 7 weeks: isometrics.
VIII. 6 to 8 weeks: Initiate CPM.
IX. Up to 6 months: no lifting, jarring, pounding, pushing, or weight bearing.

REFERENCE

1. Ferlic DC: Rheumatoid arthritis in the elbow. p. 1767. In Green DP (ed): Operative Hand Surgery. 2nd Ed. Vol. 3. Churchill Livingstone, New York, 1988

SUGGESTED READINGS

Ewald FC: Operative Techniques for the Capitello-Condylar Total Elbow Prosthesis. Brigham and Women's Hospital and Harvard University Medical School, Boston, MA
Ewald FC, Jacobs MA: Total elbow arthroplasty. Clin Orthop Relat Res 182:137, 1984
Occupational Therapy Section, Good Samaritan Hospital, Baltimore, MD. Capitella-Condylar Total Elbow Replacement Protocol.

Metacarpophalangeal Joint Arthroplasty

31

Lorie Theisen

Metacarpophalangeal (MCP) joint flexible implant arthroplasty is frequently indicated for patients with rheumatoid arthritis. Pain, joint instability, and deformities are common problems. Typically, in rheumatoid arthritis, ulnar drift of the fingers and subluxation of the MCP joint occurs. Radial deviation of the metacarpals secondary to wrist malalignment is thought to cause the ulnar drift deformity. Other causes include posture, gravitational forces, and dynamic flexion forces.[1–3]

In flexible implant arthroplasty the term implant refers to a flexible silastic spacer rather than a joint. One of the main functions of the spacer is to maintain alignment and spacing during the early stages of healing and rehabilitation. Early motion is important in promoting the development of a fibrous joint capsule. The process where the implant acts as a spacer to support the newly forming fibrous capsule is the encapsulation process.[4–7] Early protected motion ensures a greater range of motion, assists in decreasing edema, promotes an organized arrangement of collagen fibers, and prevents malalignment.

DEFINITION

A surgical formation or reformation of the MCP joints, typically a flexible implant, is used (Fig. 31-1).

SURGICAL PURPOSE

To restore skeletal alignment and tendon repositioning for more effective and efficient finger function. Flexible implant arthroplasty is most commonly used for patients with rheumatoid arthritis. The surgery is also

241

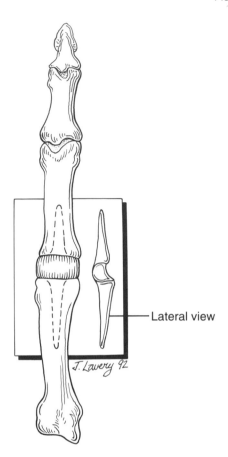

—Lateral view

J. Lavery 92

Fig. 31-1. Views of implant.

performed in cases of other types of arthritic conditions resulting from trauma, infection, or systemic diseases. The silicone implant acts primarily as a bone spacer. Soft tissue reconstruction around the joint may include collateral ligament repair and extensor tendon realignment. Postoperative therapy and monitoring is an integral part of the treatment to assure a satisfactory end result. Greatly improved appearance of the hand is also achieved.

TREATMENT GOALS

   I. Monitor wound healing
  II. Decrease edema
 III. Prevent scar adherence
 IV. Active MCP flexion to 70 degrees and extension to neutral
  V. Neutral alignment of each digit with the corresponding metacarpal
 VI. Prevent rotational deformities

POSTOPERATIVE INDICATIONS/PRECAUTIONS FOR THERAPY

I. Indications

MCP arthroplasty with flexible implant

II. Precautions

A. Extensive reconstruction of soft tissues, limited bone stock, or arthrodesis of adjacent joints may require a delay in initiating postoperative rehabilitation and may require additional protective splinting during the postoperative rehabilitation.

B. Delay in wound healing that may be due to medical conditions and/or nonsteroidal anti-inflammatory drug or steroid use.

C. Presence of osteoporosis.

D. Greater than expected postoperative pain may indicate a flare up of rheumatoid arthritis or infection.

POSTOPERATIVE THERAPY

I. 2 to 6 days postoperatively: the bulky dressing is removed and a dynamic MCP extension splint is applied over a lightly padded dressing (Fig. 31-2). The surgeon should be consulted if there is any question about the timing of the first visit. The pull of the slings is full MCP extension when at rest and appropriate tension to allow active MCP flexion. Keep in mind that the final goal is 70 degrees MCP flexion.

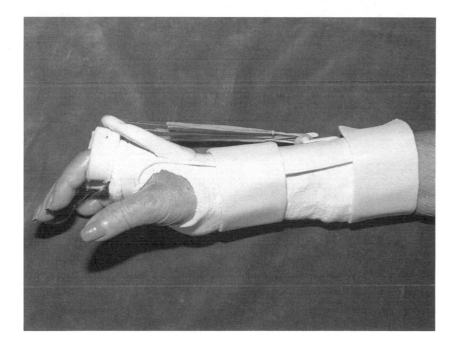

Fig. 31-2. Dynamic extension splint for postoperative treatment.

The slings should also pull in approximately 15 degrees of radial direction to prevent ulnar forces. Interphalangeal (IP) extension blocks or troughs to prevent proximal interphalangeal (PIP) flexion during active MCP flexion exercises may be applied. If the troughs are applied volarly, they should be carefully applied so that the digits are not positioned in an ulnar direction. Dorsally applied troughs may be easier to apply correctly. The dynamic splint is worn continuously (a static splint may be fabricated for night use) (Fig. 31-3) and active MCP flexion exercises intermittently throughout the waking hours.

II. 2 to 3 weeks postoperatively: MCP flexion assists (e.g., dynamic flexion splinting) may be initiated for intermittent use throughout the day. The MCP flexion splint should not pull the fingers in an ulnar direction. It is important to work diligently to obtain MCP extension and flexion goals in the first 3 weeks.[8,9]

III. 6 weeks postoperatively: dynamic MCP extension splinting is gradually tapered to night splinting only with the following exceptions:
A. Presence of MCP extension lag.
B. Presence of MCP flexion contracture.
   In these cases continue splinting for the existing deformities. Initiate appropriate activities of daily living (ADL) and education on joint protection techniques.

IV. 8 to 10 weeks: mild isometric resistive exercises may be initiated, if ulnar forces are avoided. Isometric exercises may be useful in preventing ulnar forces.

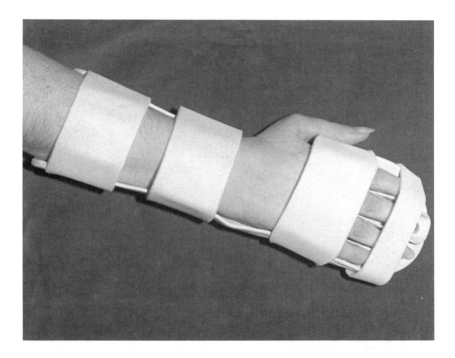

Fig. 31-3. Static positioning splint.

POSTOPERATIVE COMPLICATIONS

I. Pronation deformity or medial rotation may occur. To resolve this deformity additional outriggers to provide a rotational force at the MCP joint may be necessary. The combined pull of a force couple (force couple is two equal and opposite forces that act along parallel lines)[9] may be necessary. The force couple is obtained by applying another outrigger to the digit with a pronation tendency. The combined forces produce a force in supination direction of the digit and allow MCP extension and flexion as well.[10]

II. Extension contracture at the fifth digit may occur. Therefore, the dynamic splinting and range of motion (ROM) programs should be carefully monitored. Tension on the dynamic MP portion may need to be reduced for the fifth digit.

III. Dislocation or fracture of implant may occur.

IV. Slow healing with steroid medication (wound care precautions).

EVALUATION TIMELINE

I. 2 to 7 days postoperatively: initial assessment including active ROM measurement of the MCP joints.

II. Reassessment of ROM every week thereafter.

III. 8 to 10 weeks: Grip strength using a modified blood pressure cuff may be initiated.[11]

REFERENCES

1. Flatt A: Care of the Rheumatoid Hand. 4th Ed. CV Mosby, St. Louis, 1983

2. Smith RR, Kaplan E: Rheumatoid deformities at the MCP joints. J Bone Joint Surg 49A:31, 1967

3. Hakstan R, Tubiana R: Ulnar deviation of the fingers: the role of joint structure and function. J Bone Joint Surg 49A:299, 1967

4. Flatt AS: Restoration of rheumatoid finger joint function. J Bone Joint Surg 45A:753, 1961

5. Swanson A: Flexible implant arthroplasty for arthritis finger joints. J Bone Joint Surg 54A:435, 1972

6. Swanson A, Swanson G, Leonard J: Postoperative rehabilitation programs in flexible implant arthroplasty of the digits. p. 912. In Hunter J (ed): Rehabilitation of the Hand. 3rd Ed. CV Mosby, St. Louis, 1990

7. Leonard J, Swanson A, Swanson G: Post-operative care for patients with silastic finger joint implants. 4th Ed. Dow Corning Corporation, Midland, MI, 1985

8. Madden J, Devore G, Arem A: A rational post-operative management program for metacarpophalangeal joint implant arthroplasty. J Hand Surg 2(5): 358, 1977

9. Swanson A, Swanson G, Leonard J: Postoperative rehabilitation programs in

flexible implant arthroplasty of the digits. p. 912. In Hunter J (ed): Rehabilitation of the Hand. 3rd Ed. CV Mosby, St. Louis, 1990
10. Devore G, Muhleman C, Sasarita S: Management of pronation deformity in metacarpophalangeal joint implant arthroplasty. J Hand Surg 11A(6):859, 1986
11. Melvin J: Evaluation of muscle strength. p. 291. In: Rheumatic Disease Occupational Therapy and Rehabilitation. 2nd Ed. FA Davis, Philadelphia, 1982

SUGGESTED READINGS

Aren A, Madden J: Effects of stress on healing wounds: intermittent noncyclical tension. J Surg Res 20:93, 1976

Beckenbaugh R, Dobyns J, Linscheid R: Review and analysis of silicone–rubber metacarpophalangeal implants. J Bone Joint Surg 58A(4):483, 1976

Bieber E, Weiland A, Volence Dowling S: Silicone rubber implant arthroplasty of the metacarpophalangeal joints for rheumatoid arthritis. J Bone Joint Surg 68A(2)206, 1986

Bryant M: Wound healing. Clin Symp Ciba Ser 29(3):2, Summit, NJ, 1977

Ehrlich G: Rehabilitation Management of Rheumatic Conditions. 2nd Ed. Williams & Wilkins, Baltimore, 1986

Gardner R, Mowat A: Wound healing after operations on patients with rheumatoid arthritis. J Bone Joint Surg 55B(1):134, 1973

Kloth L, McCulloch J, Feedar J: Wound Healing: Alternatives in Management. FA Davis, Philadelphia, 1990

Melvin J: Rheumatic Disease in the Adult and Child. 3rd Ed. FA Davis, Philadelphia, 1982

Utsinger P, Zuaifler N, Ehrlich G: Rheumatoid Arthritis Etiology, Diagnosis, and Management. JB Lippincott, Philadelphia, 1989

Vahuanen V, Viljakka T: Silicone rubber implant arthroplasty of the metacarpophalangeal joint in rheumatoid arthritis: a follow-up study of 32 patients. J Hand Surg 11A(3):333, 1986

Proximal Interphalangeal and Distal Interphalangeal Joint Arthroplasty

32

Lorie Theisen

Flexible implant arthroplasty may be indicated for the proximal inter-phalangeal (PIP) or the distal interphalangeal (DIP) joints of the digits. PIP or DIP joint arthroplasty is indicated in the presence of pain, stiffness, deformities, instability about a joint, and loss of cartilage. These findings may be a sequelae of osteoarthritis, rheumatoid arthritis, or trauma (Fig. 32-1).

An acceptable alternative procedure to flexible implant arthroplasty of the distal joints is arthrodesis. The advantages and disadvantages of each procedure are weighed carefully by the surgeon. Since hand function is significantly limited by a decrease in range of motion (ROM) at the PIP joints, particularly of the ulnar fingers, arthroplasty of the PIP joint is often preferred over arthrodesis. Hand function is only minimally limited by a decrease in DIP joint ROM; therefore, arthrodesis is often preferred at the DIP joint. Arthroplasty of the DIP joint is indicated where ROM as well as pain relief is necessary.

DEFINITION

A surgical formation or reformation of the PIP or DIP joints

SURGICAL PURPOSE

The surgical management of acquired or post-traumatic arthritis of the PIP or DIP joints can improve function and joint alignment. Two basic types of arthroplasty can be employed: silastic joint spacers or a soft tissue interpositional joint spacer. Relief of pain and improvement of joint motion is of primary importance in undertaking these operations.

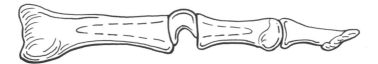

Fig. 32-1. Flexible implant arthroplasty of a PIP joint.

TREATMENT GOALS

The usual postoperative treatment goals regarding wound healing, edema control, and scar management apply. The encapsulated process and associated rehabilitation principles described in postoperative guidelines for metacarpophalangeal (MCP) joint arthroplasty also apply. Specifically, following PIP arthroplasty of the ring and small fingers the goal is pain-free active ROM (AROM) to 70 degrees flexion and neutral extension. For the index and middle fingers, less flexion is acceptable. Following DIP arthroplasty the goal is 30 degrees flexion and neutral extension. Tendencies toward deformities such as boutonniere or swan neck should be addressed. Finally, the surgeon should be contacted if there is any question regarding joint stability and progression of the mobilization phase of rehabilitation.

POSTOPERATIVE INDICATIONS/PRECAUTIONS FOR THERAPY

I. Indications
    A. Rehabilitation is indicated following surgical reformation of a joint and surgical implant of a flexible silastic spacer.
II. Precautions
    A. The initiation of the remobilization program is dependent on the stability of the joint. Consult the physician regarding the timing of the ROM exercise program.
    B. Additional surgical procedures, such as ligament repair, tendon repositioning or reconstruction, tenolysis, or volar plate release may require adherence to additional rehabilitation principles and precautions.

POSTOPERATIVE THERAPY

I. PIP arthroplasty
    A. For a preoperative stiff PIP joint requiring joint release procedures:
        1. 3 to 5 days postoperatively begin AROM of the PIP joint, avoiding any lateral deviation.
        2. Continuous static extension splinting (Fig. 32-2), except during exercise, for 6 weeks postoperatively. Alternatively, dynamic

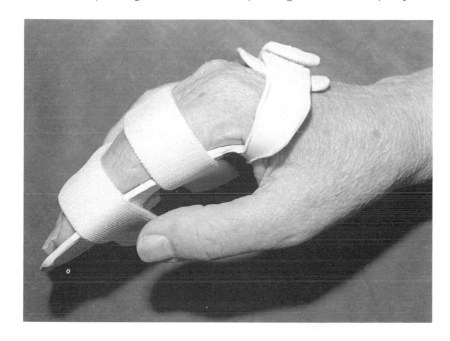

Fig. 32-2. Static PIP extension splint may be used following arthroplasty for a stiff PIP joint.

PIP extension splinting with intermittent active flexion in the splint may be used. The dynamic splint should be designed to control lateral forces (Fig. 32-3).

3. Dynamic flexion splinting, to gain 70 degrees, may be initiated after the third week postoperatively (Fig. 32-4).

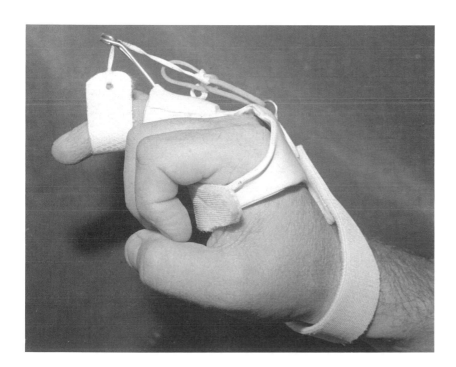

Fig. 32-3. Dynamic PIP extension splint may be used following arthroplasty for a stiff PIP joint.

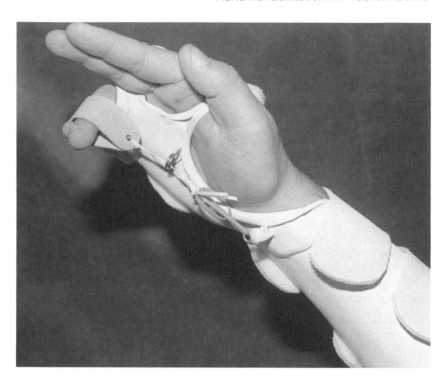

Fig. 32-4. Dynamic flexion splinting may be used to improve PIP flexion.

B. For a boutonnière deformity, the main goal is to maintain PIP extension and DIP flexion.
  1. Maintain static protective splinting with the PIP joint in full extension and continue for 3 to 6 weeks postoperatively. Active DIP flexion exercises with the PIP joint extended are indicated to maintain the oblique retinacular ligament length.
  2. 10 to 14 days postoperatively: active flexion and extension exercises of the PIP joint are initiated with the MCP joint in extension. Static extension splinting continues with intermittent AROM exercises up to 10 weeks postoperatively.
  3. Buddy splinting may be indicated to protect against lateral forces (Fig. 32-5).
C. For a swan-neck deformity the main goal during the postoperative rehabilitation process is to maintain PIP flexion and DIP extension.
  1. 0 to 10 days postoperatively: continue digital static extension splinting with the PIP in 10 degrees to 20 degrees of flexion and DIP in full extension.
  2. 10 to 14 days postoperatively: initiate AROM. During exercise maintain 10 degrees of flexion at the PIP joint, and avoid extreme flexion at the DIP joint.
  3. 14 days postoperatively: initiate gentle passive exercises in flexion and extension.[1,2]

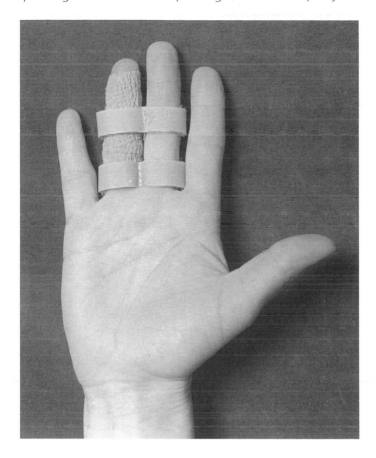

Fig. 32-5. Buddy splint may be used following arthroplasty for a boutonniere deformity.

II. DIP arthroplasty
   A. Without Kirschner wire (K-wire) fixation.
      1. PIP and DIP joints are in extension for 2 weeks.
      2. DIP joint is held in extension for an additional 2 weeks and PIP joint AROM is initiated.
      3. Gentle active flexion is initiated after this immobilization period. Flexion should be performed gradually, progressing to 30 degrees of flexion. Night extension splinting continues for an additional 6 weeks.
   B. With K-wire fixation.
      1. 3 to 4 weeks of fixation followed by an additional 4 weeks of DIP extension splinting (Fig. 32-6).
      2. Gradual AROM to 30 degrees of DIP flexion may be initiated after removal of fixation.
      3. Night DIP extension splinting for another 2 months.
III. Adjunctive treatment
   Consider the use of a continuous passive movement (CPM) unit as an adjunct to treatment.

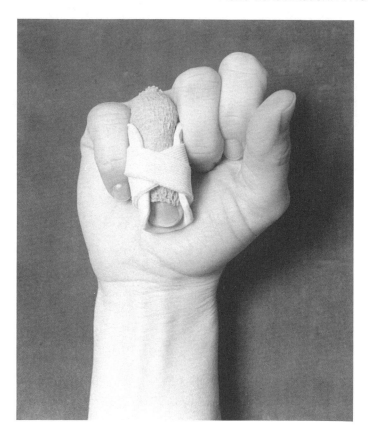

Fig. 32-6. DIP extension splinting follows K-wire immobilization for a DIP arthroplasty.

POSTOPERATIVE COMPLICATIONS

I. PIP arthroplasty
   A. Flexor tendon adherence
   B. Malalignment
   C. Extension lag
   D. Fracture of the prosthesis
   E. Synovitis
II. DIP arthroplasty
   A. Malalignment
   B. Mallet finger
   C. Fracture of the prosthesis
   D. Synovitis

EVALUATION TIMELINE

I. PIP arthroplasty
   A. 3 to 5 days postoperatively: initial AROM measurements.
   B. Re-evaluation every 2 weeks thereafter.

    C. Strength measurements once joint stability is well established. A modified blood pressure cuff may be indicated for strength testing.[3]

II. DIP arthroplasty

    A. 4 weeks postoperatively: Initial AROM measurements

    B. Re-evaluation every 2 weeks thereafter

    C. Strength measurements once joint stability is well established. A modified blood pressure cuff for testing may be indicated.

REFERENCES

1. Swanson AB, Swanson-deGroot G, Leonard J: Post-operative rehabilitation programs in flexible implant arthroplasty of the digits. p. 133, 142. In Hunter J (ed): Rehabilitation of the Hand. 2nd Ed. CV Mosby, St. Louis, 1984
2. Swanson AB, Maupin BK, Gajjar NV: Flexible implant arthroplasty in the proximal interphalangeal joint of the hand. J Hand Surg 10A:796, 1985
3. Melvin JL: Evaluation of muscle strength. p. 291. In: Surgical Rehabilitation, Rheumatic Disease Occupational Therapy and Rehabilitation. 2nd Ed. FA Davis, Philadelphia, 1982

SUGGESTED READINGS

Beckenbaugh RD, Linscheid RL: Arthroplasty in the hand and wrist. p. 167. In Green DP (ed): Operative Hand Surgery. 2nd Ed. Vol. 1. Churchill Livingstone, New York, 1988

Milford L: Reconstruction after injury. p. 283. In: Campbell's Operative Orthopaedics. 7th Ed. Vol. 1. CV Mosby, St. Louis, 1987

Pellegrini D, Burton R: Osteoarthritis of the proximal interphalangeal joint of the hand: arthroplasty or fusion? J Hand Surg 15A:194, 1990

Smith RJ: Balance of kinetics of the fingers under normal pathological conditions. Clin Orthop Relat Res 104:92, 1974

Swanson AB, Swanson-deGroot G: Treatment Considerations and Resource Materials for Flexible (Silicone) Implant Arthroplasty. Orthopedic Research Dept., Blodgett Memorial Medical Center, Grand Rapids, 1987

Swanson AB, Swanson deGroot G: Postoperative Care for Patients with Silastic Finger Joint Implants (Swanson Design). 4th Ed. Orthopaedic Reconstructive Surgeons P.C., Grand Rapids, 1985

Zimmerman NB, Shuhey PV, Clark GL, Wilgis EFS: Silicone Interpositional Arthroplasty of the Distal Interphalangeal Joint. J Hand Surg 14A:882, 1989

Thumb Carpometacarpal Joint Arthroplasty

33

Rebecca J. Gorman

Basal joint arthroplasty is indicated when there is significant arthritis of the trapezio–metacarpal joint and/or adjacent joints of the thumb, which results in disabling pain and loss of hand function. Surgical intervention may be necessary if the patient fails to respond to a conservative management regime of splinting, nonseroidal anti-inflammatories, and/or steroid injection. Some authors advocate strengthening exercises for the "muscles of the thenar cone as well as the extrinsic abductor, long extensor, and long flexor."[1] Arthritic changes can be degenerative, traumatic, or due to systemic disease as in rheumatoid arthritis. Disease of the thumb carpometacarpal (CMC) joint occurs more frequently in women than in men, and is thought to be related to activities that require "continuous tone in the thenar musculature during thumb flexion–adduction."[2]

Surgical options in basal joint arthroplasty include silicone implant or soft tissue reconstruction. Implant arthroplasty is usually reserved for the relatively low demand rheumatoid hand due to the potential complications of silicone synovitis and/or subluxation. There are many different types of soft tissue reconstructions performed and the following protocol is based on the Burton–Pellegrini procedure. Range of motion (ROM) after this procedure is approximately the same as it was prior to surgery. Functionally, a slight decrease in grip and pinch strength is to be expected due to the slight shortening of the first ray despite the fact that these functions are now less painful.[3] As with any surgical procedure involving the hand, close communication with the surgeon is necessary to facilitate complete patient care.

DEFINITION

The trapezium is excised and the base of the first metacarpal is resected. A soft tissue spacer is constructed from either the palmaris longus or part of the flexor carpi radialis (FCR) and inserted in the trapezial space; then the joint capsule is closed. Ligamentous stability is often augmented by taking part of the FCR through a drill hole in the first metacarpal and then suturing it back on itself. The abductor pollicis longus tendon is also sometimes imbricated to increase stability (Fig. 33-1).

SURGICAL PURPOSE

Surgical correction of arthritis of the carpometacarpal joint of the thumb is designed mainly to relieve pain. Secondary gains are the improved positioning of the thumb with greater active range of motion (AROM) due to the decreased pain. This provides better thumb function and appearance. When there is secondary deformity of the metacarpophalangeal (MCP) joint, it may also have to be surgically corrected.

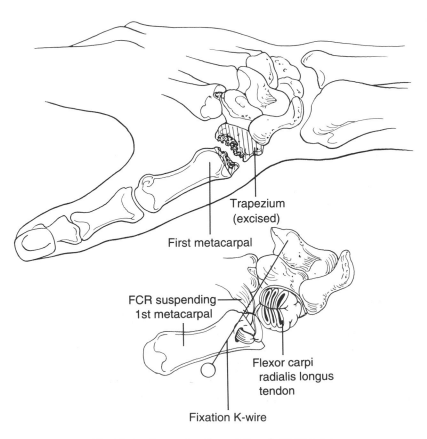

Trapezium
(excised)

First metacarpal

FCR suspending
1st metacarpal

Flexor carpi
radialis longus
tendon

Fixation K-wire

Fig. 33-1. Reconstruction of thumb CMC joint.

TREATMENT GOALS

I. Edema control
II. Pain control
III. Increase ROM, strength, and functional use of the hand
IV. Promotion of a stable, mobile, and pain-free joint

POSTOPERATIVE INDICATIONS/PRECAUTIONS FOR THERAPY

MCP joint hyperextension can be a concurrent problem and this may necessitate additional surgical procedures such as MCP fusion or capsulodesis. Consult the operative note when possible.

POSTOPERATIVE THERAPY

I. 0 to 2 weeks
   A. The patient is immobilized in a thumb spica cast.
II. 2 to 4 weeks
   A. The bulky, postoperative dressing and sutures are removed and the use of elastic stockinette or Coban can be initiated for edema control.
   B. The patient is fitted with a thumb spica cast or splint with the interphalangeal (IP) joint left free for ROM (Fig. 33-2).
   C. The cast or splint is used continuously until the initiation of active ROM (AROM) of the CMC at 4 to 6 weeks postoperatively.

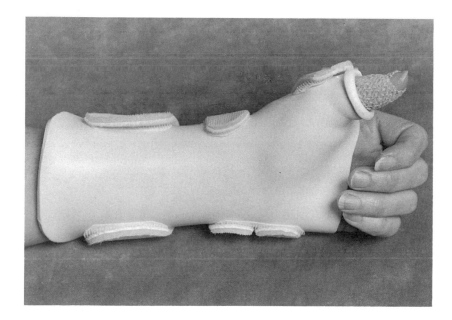

Fig. 33-2. Coban used for edema control may be worn with a thumb spica splint.

III. 4 to 6 weeks
   A. Active assistive ROM and AROM are initiated to the thumb and
      wrist.
   B. Exercises should emphasize abduction, extension, and opposi-
      tion to each fingertip.
   C. Early metacarpal flexion and adduction puts undue stress on the
      reconstructed ligament and should be minimized at this time.
   D. Complete flexion across the palm to the base of the fifth metacar-
      pal should not be attempted until the thumb can oppose each
      fingertip with ease, and gradually be worked down to the base of
      the small finger.[2]
   E. Splinting is continued after exercise and at night primarily for
      patient comfort.
IV. 7 weeks
   Dynamic splinting to increase MCP and IP joint motion can be
   initiated if the CMC joint is well stabilized.
 V. 8 to 10 weeks
   A. Static splint use can be discontinued if the joint is stable and
      patient is asymptomatic.
   B. Gentle strengthening including grip and pinch strengthening can
      be initiated if the joint is stable and relatively pain free.[4]
VI. 10 to 12 weeks
   Normal use of the hand may be resumed without restrictions pro-
   vided the joint is stable and the patient is asymptomatic.

POSTOPERATIVE COMPLICATIONS

 I. The carpal tunnel is in close proximity to the basal joint and postoper-
    ative edema can exacerbate an underlying median nerve problem
    or cause an acute carpal tunnel. This responds well to conservative
    management. If a concurrent carpal tunnel release was performed the
    patient may take longer to regain strength.
 II. DeQuervain's syndrome may become symptomatic during therapy.
    If recognized, it responds well to conservative treatment, including
    splinting, nonsteroidal anti-inflammatory drugs, and/or injection.[3]
III. Hypersensitivity of the thenar region and incisional area is not an
    uncommon complication and when present needs to be treated with
    desensitization and pain control techniques. The therapist should be
    on the alert for signs and symptoms of reflex sympathetic dystrophy
    (RSD), as prompt diagnosis and early intervention is the most effective
    treatment for this disabling disease.

EVALUATION TIMELINE

 I. Preoperative evaluation, when possible, should include:
   A. ROM
   B. Grip and pinch strength
   C. Sensation

II. Postoperative evaluation
  A. 2 weeks
    1. Blocked active and passive MCP and IP ROM
  B. 4 weeks
    1. MCP and IP ROM
    2. CMC abduction and extension
    3. Opposition, active only
    4. Wrist ROM
  C. 8 weeks
    1. Thumb ROM (CMC, MCP, IP)
    2. Wrist ROM
    3. Grip and pinch strength (providing the CMC joint is stable and the patient is asymptomatic)
    4. Sensation

REFERENCES

1. Burton R: Basal joint implant arthroplasty in osteoarthritis. Hand Clin 3(4): 473, 1987
2. Burton R: Complications following surgery on the basal joint of the thumb. Hand Clin 2(2):265, 1986
3. Eaton R: Trapezometacarpal osteoarthritis staging as a rationale for treatment. Hand Clin 3(4):455, 1987
4. Cannon NM, Eaton R, Glickel S (eds): Soft tissue reconstructions CMC joint. Diagnosis and Treatment Manual for Physicians and Therapists. 3rd Ed. Hand Rehabilitation Center of Indiana PC, Indianapolis, 1991

SUGGESTED READINGS

Amadio P, Millender L, Smith R: Silicone spacer or tendon spacer for trapezium, resection arthroplasty—comparison of results. J Hand Surg 7(3):237, 1982

Burton R, Pellegrini V: Surgical management of basal joint arthritis of the thumb. Part II. Ligament reconstruction with tendon interposition arthroplasty. J Hand Surg 11A(3):324, 1986

Eaton R, Glickel S, Littler W: Tendon interposition arthroplasty for degenerative arthritis of the trapeziometacarpal joint of the thumb. J Hand Surg 10A(5):645, 1985

Froimson A: Tendon interposition arthroplasty of carpometacarpal joint of the thumb. Hand Clin 3(4), 1987

Ulnar Collateral Ligament Injury of the Thumb

34

Arlynne Pack Brown

The function of the thumb metacarpophalangeal (MCP) joint is dependent on the stability rather than the mobility of this joint.[1] Progression through all rehabilitation procedures should be based on continual reassessment of the stability of the ulnar aspect of the joint.

Ulnar collateral joint ligament (UCL) injuries to the thumb MCP joints can be divided into two categories for the purposes of rehabilitation. One category consists of incomplete ligament tears and nondisplaced bony avulsions treated with immobilization. The other category consists of complete tears and displaced bony avulsions treated with surgery and immobilization.

The major distinction between partial and complete ligament tears is the likelihood for complete tears to become Stener lesions. Stener lesions are formed by avulsed ligaments sliding out from under the adductor aponeurosis and flipping on top of the adductor aponeurosis. These lesions require surgical repair to restore lateral stability. Conversely, if the ligament is partially torn and the joint demonstrates minimal instability, the joint can be immobilized in plaster. The surgeon may position the joint in slight flexion and ulnar deviation to assure stability (Fig. 34-1).

Rehabilitation for the two categories follows identical progression with exception of the amount of time the joint is immobilized. According to the literature noted in the attached bibliography, incomplete ligament tears and nondisplaced avulsion fractures are immobilized for 3 to 6 weeks. Surgically repaired injuries are immobilized for 4 to 6 weeks or longer. The precise amount of time of immobilization should be determined by the surgeon given his/her knowledge of the actual repair and subsequent expectations.

During the immobilization period the primary goal is to maintain the range of motion (ROM) of the unaffected joints. Distinct attention should be given to the thumb interphalangeal (IP) joint to prevent tendon adhesions.

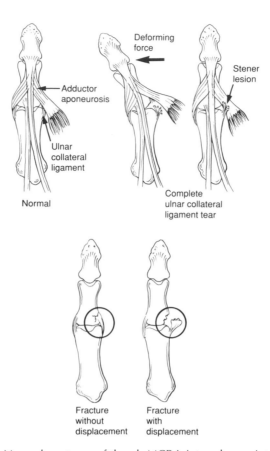

Fig. 34-1. Normal anatomy of thumb MCP joint and associated injuries.

Once the splint is removed, active ROM (AROM) is initiated. Following this, passive ROM (PROM) and dynamic splinting will begin in 1-week increments of time.

Gentle, resistive strengthening for partial tears may begin at status post 8 weeks and for repaired complete tears at 10 to 12 weeks. Unrestricted activities for partial tears may begin at 10 to 16 weeks and for repaired complete tears at 12 to 16 weeks.

DEFINITION

  I. Incomplete tears of UCL: partial tears of UCL with minimal lateral instability

 II. Nondisplaced bony avulsions: injury to bone at attachment of UCL without displacement

III. Complete tear of UCL.
   A. Stener lesions: complete UCL tears *with* adductor pollicis tendon interpositioning
   B. Complete UCL tears *without* adductor pollicis tendon interpositioning
   C. Displaced avulsion fractures
IV. Other names for UCL injuries
   A. Gamekeeper's thumb
   B. Skier's thumb
   C. Stener's lesion
   D. Breakdancer's thumb

TREATMENT PURPOSE

The UCL of the thumb MCP joint stabilizes that joint against forces applied in a radial direction to the thumb. If the ligament's integrity is lost, the thumb tends to "run away" from the index finger and the power of pinch is significantly reduced. The treatment protocol depends on the consideration of how much of this ligament is torn and how unstable the joint may become. The management ranges on the treatment scale from simple splinting, to operative repair including fracture fixation. The goal is to recognize the extent of the injury very early and begin appropriate care.

Late reconstruction can seriously compromise the stability and ROM of the thumb MCP joint when compared with normal.

TREATMENT GOALS

   I. Maintain full ROM of all uninvolved joints of the upper extremity
   II. Promote ligament healing
   III. Avoid pin tract and/or pullout wire tract infection
   IV. Maximize MCP joint AROM and PROM
   V. Maximize lateral stability of MCP joint during grip and pinch activities
   VI. Return to previous level of function
   VII. Prevent re-injury

NONOPERATIVE INDICATIONS/PRECAUTIONS FOR THERAPY

I. Indications
   A. Incomplete UCL tears
   B. Nondisplaced bony avulsions at site of UCL attachment
II. Precautions
   A. Avoid torque, which would further tear UCL

B. Extreme pain

C. Extreme edema

D. Associated flexor or extensor tendon ruptures

NONOPERATIVE THERAPY

Following incomplete UCL tears or nondisplaced avulsion fractures

I. Weeks 1 through 3 to 6: thumb spica plaster or thermoplastic splint immobilization for amount of time directed by surgeon.[1-4] Consult surgeon as to whether immobilization of the IP and wrist joints is indicated (Fig. 34-2).

Maintain AROM of all joints of the upper extremity while in plaster/splint. Concentrate especially on the IP joint to prevent extensor mechanism adhesions.

II. Week 4: If splint includes the wrist (forearm based), cut it down to exclude the wrist (hand based). Wear splint while sleeping, in crowds, and other tenuous situations.

Initiate AROM of the MCP joint.

III. Week 5: Begin and progress PROM of the thumb MCP joint.

IV. Week 6: Begin and progress dynamic splinting of the thumb MCP joint as needed.

V. Week 8: Begin and progress strengthening especially of the structures on the ulnar border of the joint, during grip and pinch. Specifically, strengthen the locking of the thumb around a 6 to 8 cm diameter cylinder.[5,6] Strengthening muscles for pinch in lateral, tip, and three jaw positions (Fig. 34-3).

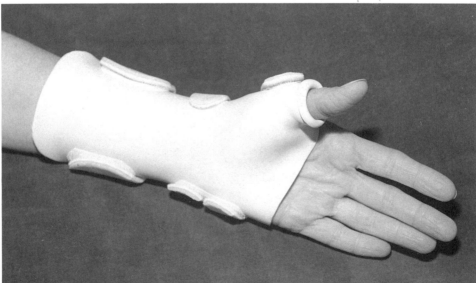

Fig. 34-2. Example of postoperative thumb splint.

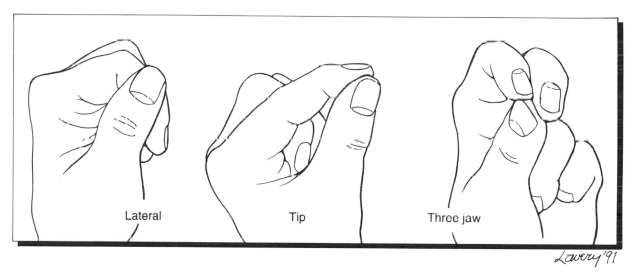

Fig. 34-3. Pinch positions.

VI. Weeks 10 to 16: Begin unrestricted use. May want to tape protectively during sports activities.[7]

NONOPERATIVE COMPLICATIONS

   I. Chronic instability and weakness of pinch.[2,8]
  II. Persistent pain and arthritis.[3,8]
 III. Decreased ROM of MCP and IP joints.[8]

Concerns

POSTOPERATIVE INDICATIONS/PRECAUTIONS FOR THERAPY

  I. Indications
    A. Complete UCL tears
    B. Displaced avulsion fractures at site of UCL attachment
 II. Precautions
    A. Avoid torque to further tear UCL
    B. Infection
    C. Extreme pain
    D. Extreme edema
    E. Associated flexor or extensor tendon ruptures

POSTOPERATIVE THERAPY

Following surgical repair and Kirschner wiring/pull out wiring
  I. Weeks 1 through 4 to 6: Refer to section on treatment following incomplete UCL tears.

II. Week 4: If surgeon removes cast, Kirschner wire (K-wire) and pull out wire, apply hand based thumb splint. Continue splint full time except for supervised ROM of carpometacarpal and wrist joints.

III. Week 6: Begin AROM of MCP joint.[4] Protect lateral stability. Splint while sleeping, in crowds, and other tenuous situations.

IV. Week 7 to 8: Begin gentle PROM of MCP joint.

V. Weeks 8 to 10: Begin and progress dynamic splinting of the MCP joint if indicated.

VI. Weeks 10 to 12: Begin and progress strengthening, especially of the structures on the ulnar border during grip and pinch. Specifically, strengthen the locking of the thumb around a 6 to 8 cm diameter cylinder.[5,6] Plus, strengthening the muscles for pinch in lateral, tip, and three jaw positions.

VII. Weeks 12 to 16: Begin unrestricted use.[7] May want to tape protectively during sports activities.[4]

POSTOPERATIVE COMPLICATIONS

I. Chronic instability and weakness of pinch.[2,8]
II. Persistent numbness ulnar aspect of thumb.[8]
III. Persistent pain and arthritis.[3,8]
IV. Decreased ROM of MCP and IP joints.[8]
V. Infection

EVALUATION TIMELINE

I. Incomplete UCL tears.
   A. Week 1: AROM and PROM of all upper extremity joints not included in splint, except thumb and wrist
   B. Week 4: AROM thumb and wrist joints
   C. Week 5: PROM thumb and wrist joints
   D. Week 8: Grip strength and pinch strength, manual muscle testing (MMT) thumb muscles
II. UCL tears or nondisplaced avulsion fractures
   A. Weeks 1 to 3: same as incomplete UCL tears
   B. Week 6: AROM thumb joints
   C. Week 7: PROM thumb joints
   D. Week 10: grip strength, pinch strength, MMT thumb muscles

REFERENCES

1. Miller RJ: Dislocations and fracture dislocations of the metacarpophalangeal joint of the thumb. Hand Clin (4)1:45, 1988
2. Eaton RG: Injuries of the metacarpophalangeal joint of the thumb. p. 887. In Tubiana R (ed): The Hand. Vol. III, WB Saunders, Philadelphia, 1988

3. Sandzen SC: The Hand and Wrist. Williams & Wilkins, Baltimore, 1985
4. Green DP: Operative Hand Surgery. 2nd Ed. Churchill Livingstone, New York, 1988
5. Kopandji IA: Biomechanics of the thumb. p. 404. In Tubiana R (ed): The Hand. Vol. III. WB Saunders, Philadelphia, 1988
6. Aubriot JH: Injuries of the metacarpophalangeal joint of the thumb. p. 184. In Tubiana R (ed): The Hand. Vol. III. WB Saunders, Philadelphia, 1988
7. Gieck JH, Maxer V: Protective splinting for the hand and wrist. Clin Sports Med (5)4:795, 1986
8. Helm RH: Hand function after injuries to the collateral ligaments of the metacarpophalangeal joint of the thumb. J Hand Surg (12)2:252, 1987

SUGGESTED READINGS

Bowers WH: Sprains and joint injuries in the hand. Hand Clin (2)1:93, 1986
Eaton RG: Joint Injuries of the Hand. Charles C. Thomas, Springfield, 1971
Fess EE, Gettle KS, Strickland JW: Hand splinting principles and methods. CV Mosby, St. Louis, 1981
Flynn JE: Hand Surgery. 3rd Ed. Williams & Wilkins, Baltimore, 1982
Jupiter JB, Sheppard JE: Tension wire fixation of avulsion fractures of the hand. Clin Orthop Relat Res 214:113, 1987
Milford L: The Hand. CV Mosby, St. Louis, 1982
Stener B: Acute injuries to the metacarpophalangeal joint of the thumb. p. 895. In Tubiana R (ed): The Hand. Vol. III. WB Saunders, Philadelphia, 1988
Weeks PM: Management of acute hand injuries. 2nd Ed. CV Mosby, St. Louis, 1978

Proximal Interphalangeal Joint Fracture Dislocation

35

Arlynne Pack Brown

Proximal interphalangeal (PIP) joint fracture dislocations are produced through axial compression on semi-flexed or hyperextended digits. These forces usually result in dorsal dislocations and less commonly in volar dislocations.

PIP joint dislocations are described by two separate classification systems described by Eaton[1] and Bowers.[1] Regardless to which classification system subscribed, fragments less than 30 percent of the articular surface are usually stable and managed with closed reduction techniques. Those joints with greater than 30 percent of the articular surface involved are usually unstable and require management with open reduction internal fixation techniques.

Stable joints are either secured with buddy tape to the appropriate adjacent digit or protected with an extension block splint or with a combination of both techniques. Active exercises are begun 3 weeks after injury and 1 week later progressed to passive exercises and dynamic splinting. Protective buddy splinting continues as indicated. Strengthening is progressed from approximately 4 weeks after injury while monitoring stability, edema, and pain.

Unstable joints can be managed using a variety of techniques ranging in complexity from closed reduction and volar plate arthroplasty to force couple splints and progressive dynamic traction splinting. The postoperative therapy for each technique is distinct and detailed below.

Possible complications for all PIP joint dislocations are the same for all methods of treatment: recurrent subluxations, infections, limited range of motion (ROM), traumatic arthritis, and adherence of extensor tendons.

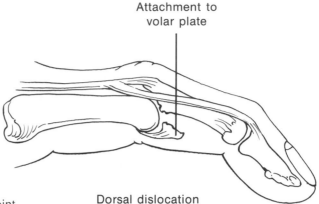

Attachment to
volar plate

Fig. 35-1. Dorsal dislocation of PIP joint.   Dorsal dislocation

DEFINITION

I. Dorsal dislocation: Middle phalanx moves dorsal in relation to proximal phalanx[1-3] (Fig. 35-1).
II. Volar dislocation: Middle phalanx moves volar in relation to proximal phalanx. This is an uncommon injury that can present clinically as a boutonniere deformity (Fig. 35-2).

TREATMENT PURPOSE

To restore maximum active ROM (AROM) to the involved joint. The surgical techniques used to achieve the reduction of the fracture with dislocation vary with the surgeon's preferences and skills. The goal is to restore the joint surfaces as accurately as possible. This may require bone grafting using the distal radius as a donor site. The type of fixation may or may not allow joint motion. Several forms of traction (or distraction) devices are used. It is extremely important for the therapist to discuss

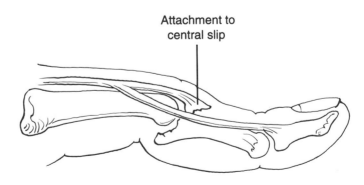

Attachment to
central slip

Fig. 35-2. Volar dislocation of PIP joint.   Volar dislocation

with the surgeon his operative technique and plans for therapy. Close monitoring of each patient's individual care is mandatory for a good final result.

TREATMENT GOALS

I. Promote maximum ROM
II. Minimize scarring
III. Prevent PIP joint flexion contracture
IV. Prevent recurrence of dislocation

NONOPERATIVE INDICATIONS/PRECAUTIONS FOR THERAPY

I. Indications
   A. PIP joint fracture dislocation treated with closed reduction, buddy taping, and/or extension block splinting
II. Precautions
   A. Unstable reduction

NONOPERATIVE THERAPY

Stable closed reduction (excluding volar plate arthroplasty)
Weeks 0 to 3: buddy tape to appropriate adjacent digit (e.g., to radial digit if radial collateral ligament tear) (Fig. 35-3)
dorsal extension block splint (Fig. 35-4)
OR
combination buddy tape and dorsal extension block splint
AROM into full flexion and to limits of extension block splint[1]
Extension block splint options.[1]

I. Tape alumifoam to proximal phalanx and limit extension to 25 degrees to 30 degrees.
II. Hand based splint with extension block incorporated.
III. Depending upon patient reliability and compliance, include block in a plaster cast/splint positioning wrist 30 degrees - 40 degrees extension, metacarpophalangeal (MCP) joints 90 degrees flexion, PIP joint 25 degrees. Remember to tape to proximal phalanx to avoid rupture of central slip.[1,3-5]
IV. If required greater than 30 degrees PIP joint flexion to maintain stability initially, then decrease flexion by 25 percent each week.[6]

Week 3: Remove extension block splint.[4]
Continue buddy taping and AROM.
Week 4: Begin dynamic extension splint.[1]

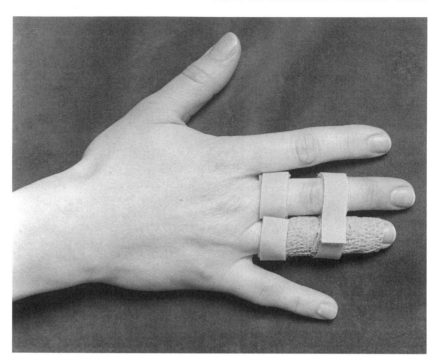

Fig. 35-3. Buddy tape to appropriate digit.

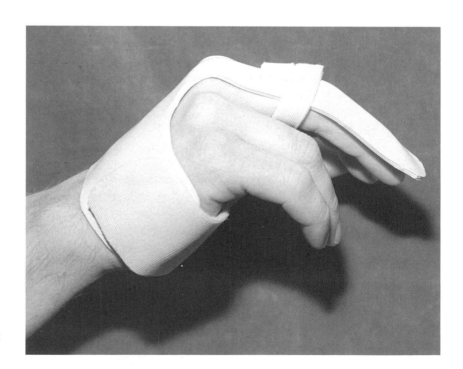

Fig. 35-4. Dorsal extension block splint.

NONOPERATIVE COMPLICATIONS

I. Progress to subluxation
II. Loss of PIP joint ROM
III. Permanent joint stiffness

POSTOPERATIVE INDICATIONS/PRECAUTIONS FOR THERAPY

I. Indications
   A. PIP joint fracture dislocation treated with open reduction internal fixation, Eaton volar plate arthroplasty, or Agee force couple traction splint
II. Precautions
   A. Unstable reduction
   B. Epiphyseal plate fractures
   C. Internal or external fixation

POSTOPERATIVE THERAPY

I. Unstable closed reduction or volar plate arthroplasty
   A. Weeks 0 to 2: Immobilize with Kirschner wire (K-wire).
   B. Weeks 2 or 3: K-wire removal by surgeon.
      1. Begin extension block splint 25 degrees.
      2. Begin AROM to limit of splint.
   C. Week 3: pull out wire removed by surgeon. Begin active extension.
   D. Week 4: Begin dynamic extension splinting with surgeon's approval. Begin light work with buddy taping.
II. Unstable acute fracture dislocations managed with Agee force couple splint (Fig. 35-5).
   A. Day 0 to 2: soft dressing
   B. Day 2: discontinue dressing. Begin antibiotic ointment to pin sites. Begin AROM exercises. Follow "unstable closed reduction or volar plate arthroplasty" guidelines after force couple splint removed by surgeon.
III. Dynamic traction splinting and early passive ROM[7] (PROM) (Fig. 35-6)
   A. Weeks 0 to 3: Wear splint continuously. Move through complete arc of ROM five times, then leave in position of extreme flexion for 2 hours alternating with extreme extension for 2 hours. Perform blocked distal interphalangeal (DIP) joint AROM.
   B. Week 3: Remove splint, begin AROM wrist. Replace splint and continue with ROM.
   C. Week 4: Begin active, blocked ROM PIP and DIP.

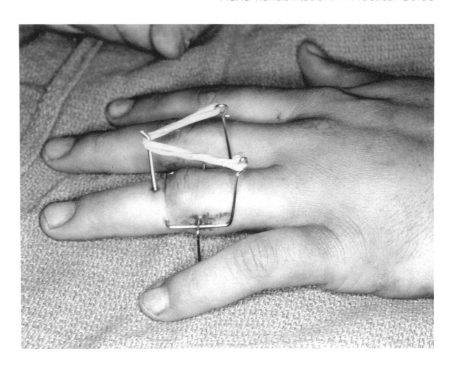

Fig. 35-5. Unstable acute fracture dislocations managed by Agee force couple splint.

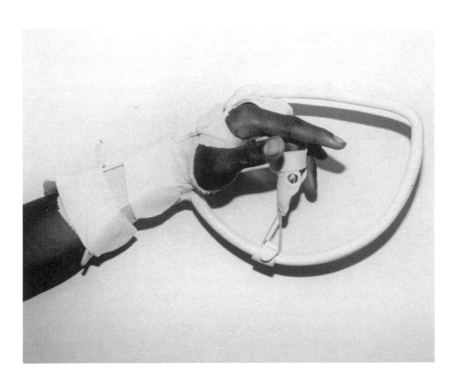

Fig. 35-6. Dynamic traction splinting allows for early PROM.

D. Week Four and one-half to 8: Remove arc splint. Fabricate protective hand based splint. Begin composite AROM.
E. Splint: basic features
   1. Molded splint extending from proximal forearm to PIP joint with wrist and MCP joints in "functional position."
   2. Modified arc with axis in line with that of PIP joint.
   3. Mold a "dutch-girl's hat" to the shape of the arc of Dowing for full arc of motion. Rubberbands attach to this arc for traction. See Schenck's 1986[7] article for more details.
   4. Amount of traction is estimated based on patient comfort and physical principles and then checked on X-ray by surgeon.

POSTOPERATIVE COMPLICATIONS

I. Recurrent subluxations[2,4]
II. Infections[2]
III. Loss of DIP joint flexion secondary to flexor tendon adhesions[2]
IV. Permanent joint stiffness[2]
V. Traumatic arthritis[2]
VI. Adherence of extensor tendon[4]

EVALUATION TIMELINE

I. Week 0 to 3
   A. Measure and begin active composite ROM to limits of extension block splint and/or buddy tape.
   B. Active blocked flexion PIP and DIP.
   C. Passive composite and blocked flexion PIP and DIP.
II. Week 3
   A. Measure and begin active composite ROM without splint.
III. Week 4
   A. Measure and begin passive composite and blocked extension ROM.
IV. Weeks 6 to 8
   A. Measure and begin grip strength.

REFERENCES

1. Lubahn JD: Dorsal fracture dislocations of the proximal interphalangeal joint. Hand Clin 4:15, 1988
2. Agee JM: Unstable fracture dislocations of the proximal interphalangeal joint. Clin Orthop Relat Res 214:101, 1987
3. Isani A: Small joint injuries requiring surgical treatment. Orthop Clin North Am 17:407, 1986
4. Eaton RG, Malerich MM: Volar plate arthroplasty of the proximal interphalangeal joint: a review of ten year's experience. J Hand Surg 5:250, 1980

5. Wilson RL, Carter MS: Joint injuries in the hand: preservation of proximal interphalangeal joint function. p. 171. In Hunter JM (ed): Rehabilitation of the Hand. 3rd. Ed. CV Mosby, Philadelphia, 1978
6. McElfresh EC, Dobyns JH, O'Brien ET: Management of fracture-dislocation of the proximal interphalangeal joints by extension block splinting. J Bone Joint Surg 54:1705, 1972
7. Schenck RR: Dynamic traction and early passive movement for fractures of the proximal interphalangeal joint. J Hand Surg 1A:850, 1986

Finger Fracture Rehabilitation

36

Gregory Hritcko

Hand fractures are a common problem and the literature indicates secondary complications frequently develop when these injuries are viewed and treated as minor.[1] Foresight and prevention are the guiding principles during the initial stages of management. Range of motion (ROM) of adjacent, noninvolved joints should be initiated as early as possible in the acute injury phase. Splint immobilization requires the intrinsic plus position of wrist extension to 30 degrees, metacarpophalangeal (MCP) joints flexed to 70 degrees to 90 degrees, and interphalangeal (IP) joints in neutral 0 degrees in order to avoid joint contractures as a result of ligament shortening. General goals of hand therapy of preserving and maximizing function apply in the initial stage as well as after fracture consolidation has been achieved. To optimize the end result, specific goals and interventions will be dictated by the type of fracture, location, degree of disruption, and management technique selected by the surgeon.

Fractures of the distal phalanx are reported as the most frequent of all hand fractures at a rate of 40 to 50 percent.[2] They most often involve the thumb and middle finger.[2] Common deformities include a tendon component (e.g., mallet finger with terminal extensor tendon avulsions and the flexor digitorum profundus avulsion fracture in the football jersey injury).

Middle phalanx fractures comprise 8 to 12 percent of hand fractures.[2] The muscle tendon units influence angulation patterns with the middle phalanx fracture. A fracture of the distal one-quarter will angulate apex volar secondary to the pull of the flexor digitorum superficialis. Proximal one-quarter fractures will commonly displace into a configuration with the apex dorsal due to the pull of the central slip of the extensor tendon. The midshaft fracture can angulate in either direction.[3,4]

Fifteen to 20 percent of hand fractures occur at the proximal phalanx level with the thumb and index finger frequently involved.[2] Midshaft proximal phalanx fractures are often spiral or oblique in configuration, which may shorten or rotate due to instability. The flexor tendon or the MCP joints may be compromised with the proximal base fracture and the proximal interphalangeal (PIP) joint may be involved with the distal neck or head fracture.[2-4]

DEFINITION

Structural break in the continuity of a bone, epiphyseal plate, or cartilaginous joint surface (Fig. 36-1)

TREATMENT PURPOSE

Fractured phalanges need to be reduced in as near normal a position as possible. Many times this can be accomplished without open reduction. If this is so, then appropriate cast or splint immobilization is required, leaving free for movement as many of the unaffected joints as possible. Open reduction is utilized to stabilize a fracture with pins or plates in order that realignment of the fragments is accomplished. The potential for early mobilization exists in these cases; however, the surgery used to accomplish the task disrupts surrounding soft tissues. These soft tissues must be considered during the healing phase. Percutaneous pinning often can achieve satisfactory fracture alignment and stabilization with minimal interference to the soft tissues. This method is often used when possible.

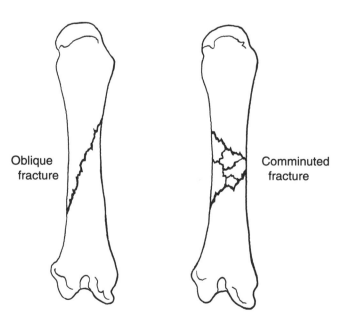

Oblique
fracture

Comminuted
fracture

Fig. 36-1. Common finger fractures are oblique and comminuted fractures.

TREATMENT GOALS

Preventative measures should be taken to preserve and maximize the function of the involved extremity. These measures should include all general goals of all hand therapy management. Specific goals will be dictated by the type of fracture, location, degree of disruption, reduction technique utilized by the surgeon, and stability of the reduction.

I. Promote healing through maintaining/protecting reduction (i.e., immobilization splint)
II. Maintain/increase ROM of noninvolved joints
III. Pain control
IV. Edema control
V. Restore and maximize the functional return of the involved extremity and joint

NONOPERATIVE INDICATIONS/PRECAUTIONS FOR THERAPY

I. Indications
   Nondisplaced fractures requiring
   A. Splinting
   B. Edema control
   C. Limited passive/active range of motion (PROM or AROM) of noninvolved joints
   D. Pain
   E. Limited PROM or AROM of involved joints
   F. Dynamic splinting
   G. Decreased strength/endurance
II. Precautions
   A. Associated concomitant soft tissue injury (neurovascular, tendon)
   B. Fracture stability, influenced by type of fracture, rate of healing, and pain level
   C. Nonunion or delayed union of fracture site

NONOPERATIVE THERAPY

I. Distal phalanx fractures
   A. Tuft fractures
      1. Protective splint to prevent re-injury, worn for 2 to 4 weeks until fracture site is nontender (Fig. 36-2).
      2. Wound care as indicated by injury mechanism.
      3. AROM begins at 2 to 4 weeks, week 0 to 1 week if fracture is stable enough.[2,3]
      4. PROM begins at 5 to 6 weeks.
      5. Strength/endurance building begins at 7 to 8 weeks.[2,3]

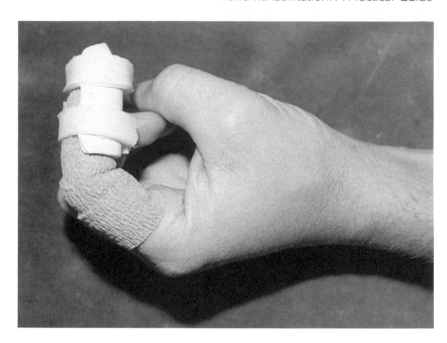

Fig. 36-2. Protective splint for a tuft fracture.

B. Shaft fractures
   1. Protective/immobilization splint worn for 3 to 4 weeks.
   2. Wound care as indicated.
   3. AROM begins at 3 to 4 weeks.
   4. PROM begins at 5 to 7 weeks.
   5. Strength/endurance building at 8 weeks.[2,3]
II. Middle phalanx fractures
    Nondisplaced
   A. Splinted in intrinsic plus position (Fig. 36-3). Immobilization should not exceed 3 weeks, avoiding PIP stiffness.[5] Buddy splinting may be a splint option requested by surgeon (Fig. 36-4).

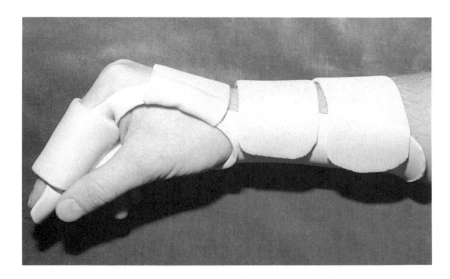

Fig. 36-3. Nondisplaced fractures may be splinted in an intrinsic plus position.

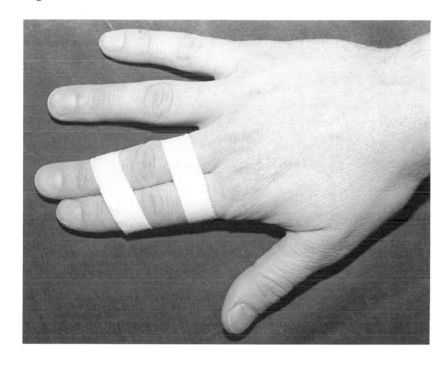

Fig. 36-4. Buddy splinting may be an option for nondisplaced fractures.

    B. AROM initiated when pain/edema subsides.
    C. 3 to 5 days for stable fracture.[3]
    D. 3 weeks for oblique or other unstable fracture.[3]
    E. PROM begins at 4 to 6 weeks.
    F. Strength/endurance building begins at 6 to 8 weeks.
III. Proximal phalanx fractures.
    A. Nondisplaced extra-articular.
       1. Splinted with buddy tape and AROM initiated immediately.[4]
       2. PROM begins at 5 to 7 weeks.[4]
       3. Strength/endurance building begins at 6 to 8 weeks.
    B. Nondisplaced intra-articular.
       1. Splinted in "intrinsic plus" position for 2 to 3 weeks.
       2. AROM begins at 2 to 3 weeks.
       3. PROM begins at 4 to 8 weeks.
       4. Strength/endurance building begins at clinical union, 8 to 12 weeks.[4]

NONOPERATIVE COMPLICATIONS

  I. Distal phalanx fracture
    A. Infection
    B. Nailbed deformities
    C. Hypersensitivity
 II. Middle phalanx fracture
    A. Tendon adhesions and decreased excursion
    B. Decreased joint mobility and stiffness[3,4]

III. Proximal phalanx fracture
   Decreased joint mobility and stiffness[3,4]
IV. General complications
   A. Infection
   B. Delayed union
   C. Malunion

POSTOPERATIVE INDICATIONS/PRECAUTIONS FOR THERAPY

I. Indications: displaced fractures requiring
   A. Splinting
   B. Edema control
   C. Limited AROM/PROM of noninvolved joints
   D. Pain
   E. Limited AROM/PROM of involved joints
   F. Dynamic splinting
   G. Decreased strength/endurance
II. Precautions
   A. Concomitant soft tissue trauma
   B. Fracture stability
   C. Nonunion or delayed union of fracture site

POSTOPERATIVE THERAPY

I. Distal phalanx fractures
   A. Shaft fractures surgically treated with percutaneous Kirschner wire (K-wire) stabilization (Fig. 36-5)
   B. Wound/pin care
   C. AROM PIP joint begins at 3 to 5 days
   D. AROM of distal interphalangeal (DIP) joint begins upon removal of K-wire at 3 to 6 weeks[2,3,6]
   E. Protective extension splinting continues for 2 to 6 additional weeks
   F. PROM initiated at 8 weeks[2,3,6]
   G. Strength/endurance building initiated at 6 to 8 weeks
II. Displaced middle phalanx fractures
   (Surgeon may select stabilizing or rigid fixation, which will guide therapy intervention.)
   A. Splinted in "intrinsic plus" position to support/protect reduction
   B. Wound/pin care
   C. AROM begins at 5 to 15 days at surgeon's recommendation; begin with gentle supported blocking exercise[4]
   D. Strength/endurance building begins at 7 to 9 weeks

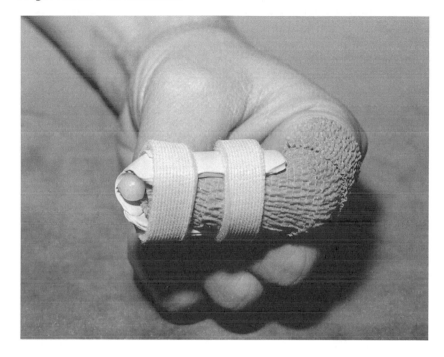

Fig. 36-5. Protective splinting for distal phalanx fracture stabilized with K-wire.

III. Displaced proximal phalanx fractures
    A. Splinted in "intrinsic plus" position
    B. Wound/pin care
    C. AROM initiated at 5 to 15 days at surgeon's recommendation and dependent upon rigid versus stabilizing fixation[4]
    D. PROM begins at 6 to 8 weeks
    E. Strength/endurance building begins at 8 to 10 weeks

POSTOPERATIVE COMPLICATIONS

  I. Distal phalanx fractures
    A. Infection
    B. Nailbed deformities
    C. Hypersensitivity
  II. Middle phalanx fractures
    A. Decreased tendon excursion and adhesions
    B. Decreased joint mobility and stiffness[3,4]
  III. Proximal phalanx fractures
    A. Associated soft tissue injuries
    B. Decreased joint mobility and stiffness[3,4]
  IV. General complications
    A. Infection
    B. Delayed union
    C. Malunion

EVALUATION TIMELINE

Appropriate baseline measures should be taken at initiation of specific exercises and repeated at 4- to 6-week intervals for documentation of progress:

I. Nonoperative

	AROM	PROM	Strength/Endurance
Distal phalanx			
Tuft fracture	2–4 weeks	5–6 weeks	7–8 weeks
Shaft fracture	3–4 weeks	5–7 weeks	8 weeks
Middle phalanx (nondisplaced)			
Stable	3–5 days	4–5 weeks	6–8 weeks
Oblique	3 weeks		
Proximal phalanx (nondisplaced)			
Extra-articular	Immediate	4–7 weeks	6–8 weeks
Intra-articular	2–3 weeks	4–5 weeks	8–12 weeks

II. Operative

	AROM	PROM	Strength/Endurance
Distal phalanx			
Shaft fracture PIP	3–5 days (postoperative)		
(With K-wire fixation) DIP	3–6 weeks (at time of K-wire removal)	8 weeks	8 weeks
Middle phalanx [displaced, open reduction, internal fixation (ORIF)]	5–15 days (postoperative)	6–8 weeks	7–9 weeks
Proximal phalanx (displaced, ORIF)	5–15 days (postoperative)	6–8 weeks	8–10 weeks

REFERENCES

1. Strickland JW, Stiechen JB, Klienman WB, Flynn M: Factors influencing digital performance after phalangeal fracture. p. 126. In Strickland JW, Stiechen JB (eds): Difficult Problems in Hand Surgery. CV Mosby, St. Louis, 1983
2. Kasch MC, Taylor-Mullins PA, Fullenwider L (eds). Hand Therapy Review Course Study Guide. Garnor, NC, 1990
3. Beasley RW: Hand Injuries. WB Saunders, Philadelphia, 1987
4. Sorenson MK: Fractures of the wrist and hand. p. 191. In Moran G (ed): Hand Rehabilitation—Clinics in Physical Therapy. Vol. 9. Churchill Livingstone, New York, 1986
5. Flynn JE: Hand Surgery. Williams & Wilkins, Baltimore, 1982

6. Connolly JF (ed): Depalma's The Management of fractures and dislocations. 3rd Ed. WB Saunders, Philadelphia, 1987

SUGGESTED READINGS

Jabaley ME, Freeland AE: Rigid internal fixation in the hand 104 cases. Plast Reconstr Surg 288, 1986

Melone CP: Rigid fixation of phalangeal and metacarpal fractures. Orthop Clin North Am 17(3):421, 1986

Packer JW, Colditz JC: Bone injuries: treatment and rehabilitation. p. 81. In Seyfor AE, Hueston JT (eds): Hand Clinics: Difficult Hand Fractures. WB Saunders, Philadelphia, 1986

Metacarpal and Proximal Interphalangeal Joint Capsulectomy

37

Rebecca J. Gorman

Capsulectomies of the metacarpophalangeal (MCP) and proximal interphalangeal (PIP) joints are performed to improve motion and functional use of stiff joints with normal articular surfaces. These procedures are necessary when stiff joints fail to respond to a conservative treatment program including splinting and exercise.

There are many anatomic structures within the finger that may limit joint motion. These structures are listed below.

I. Limited flexion (extension contracture).
   A. Scar contracture of skin over the dorsum of the finger
   B. Contracted long extensor muscle or adherent extensor tendon
   C. Contracted interosseus muscle or adherent interosseus tendon
   D. Contracted capsular ligament, particularly the collateral ligaments
   E. Bony block or exostosis
II. Limited extension
   A. Scar of skin on the volar surface of the finger
   B. Contraction of the superficial fascia in the finger, as in Dupuytren's contracture
   C. Contraction of the flexor–tendon sheath within the finger
   D. Contracted flexor muscle or adherent flexor tendon
   E. Contraction of the volar plate of the capsular ligament
   F. Adherence of the collateral ligaments with the finger in the flexed position
   G. Bony block or exostosis[1]

These multiple factors need to be evaluated clinically and at the time of surgery. Capsulectomies are frequently performed concurrently with other surgical procedures (i.e., intrinsic releases, flexor, and/or extensor tenolysis). To facilitate effective postoperative management the therapist should obtain a copy of the operative report. Curtis has stated that "the results seem to indicate that the more anatomical structures are involved in the limitation of motion, the poorer is the end result."[1]

The therapist's role in postoperative management of capsulectomies begins prior to surgery. Patient education should emphasize what will be expected of the patient postoperatively and why their postoperative performance is critical in obtaining the maximum functional benefit from the surgery.[2] As Curtis has stated, "one should not expect to restore function completely by this procedure, but one can expect to improve it."[1]

Successful management of the postcapsulectomy patient requires skillful observation, constant reassessment, and adaptation on the part of the therapist as well as a motivated and compliant patient. Maximum gains in range of motion (ROM) are usually obtained 3 to 5 months postoperatively. Patients requiring fewer surgical maneuvers, however, may continue to gain ROM for up to 6 to 8 months.[3]

DEFINITION

I. MCP capsulectomy

Surgical release of dorsal and/or volar joint capsule and collateral ligaments
II. PIP capsulectomy

Surgical release of the dorsal and/or volar joint capsule and collateral ligaments

SURGICAL PURPOSE

I. MCP capsulectomy

To restore metacarpal phalangeal joint motion where either a flexion or extension contracture exists. The capsular structures have contracted or are locally adherent to other surrounding elements (Fig. 37-1). These structures are surgically released and partially excised. Joint stability must be maintained and the passive ROM (PROM) obtained at the time of surgery is approximately the active range that can be expected with postoperative wound healing.
II. PIP capsulectomy

To restore motion to the joint that has less than a 45 degree range. The tissues surrounding the PIP joint must be considered as contributing to the contracture (e.g., skin, tendons, joint capsule, and joint surfaces) (Fig. 37-2). Tissue equilibrium (scar maturity) is essential prior to surgery. Offending scar and capsule are released or excised but joint stability is maintained. The PROM achieved at the time of surgery approximates the expected active ROM (AROM) with healing.

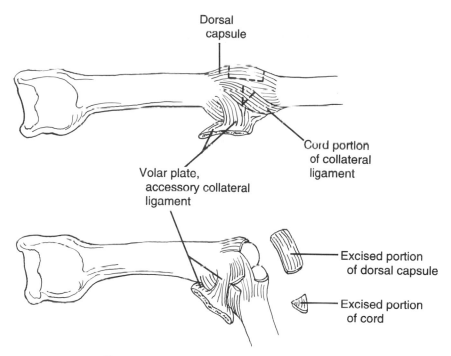

Fig. 37-1. Anatomy of MCP joint structures.

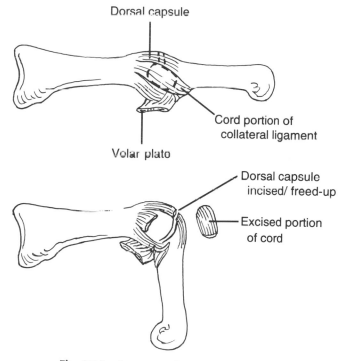

Fig. 37-2. Anatomy of PIP joint structures.

TREATMENT GOALS

I. MCP capsulectomy
    Increase PROM and AROM of the MCPs to approximately 60 degrees to 70 degrees flexion and to increase functional use of the hand.
II. PIP capsulectomy
    Restore AROM and PROM of PIP joint flexion and extension.
III. Functional goal postoperatively for both procedures: Achieve AROM equal to the PROM present after the surgical release.

POSTOPERATIVE INDICATIONS/PRECAUTIONS FOR THERAPY

I. MCP capsulectomy
    If tendons are adherent and also limiting flexion, a concurrent tenolysis may have been performed. (See the operative note.)
II. PIP capsulectomy
    This procedure is often performed in combination with other surgical procedures (i.e., tenotomy of contracted interossei, flexor, and/or extensor tenolysis). The operative report should be reviewed to ensure adequate protection and treatment of the involved anatomic structures.
    A. Precautions
        1. Intrinsic releases
            Splinting should include an intrinsic stretch splint and instruction in stretching exercises.
        2. Extensor tenolysis with volar capsulectomy secondary to flexion contracture requires dynamic extension splinting to protect the weakened and frequently stretched extensor tendon while promoting active flexion; static extension splinting is required at night.

POSTOPERATIVE THERAPY

I. General treatment principles for capsulectomies secondary to limitations of flexion and/or extension
    A. Edema control
    B. Pain management
    C. Initiation of AROM as per doctor's orders
    D. PROM, instruction in **gentle**, passive stretching
    E. Scar management
    F. Splinting
        1. It is recommended that an appointment for postoperative therapy be made when the surgery is scheduled.
        2. Dynamic splints are used during the day as an adjunct to the patient's active exercise program (and to protect weakened structures).

3. Static progressive splints are used at night to maintain gains in ROM and provide a prolonged gentle stretch to the involved soft tissues.

4. All splints need to be monitored and adjusted frequently as the soft tissues respond to the stresses applied through active and passive exercise. The patient should be provided with detailed wearing instructions and precautions.

5. Splinting is continued until the patient is able to maintain the ROM present postoperatively with AROM and PROM (approximately 3 to 5 months).

6. When passive motion exceeds active motion the emphasis on active exercise should be increased to overcome tendon weakness or adherence.

G. Functional activities and light use of the hand should be incorporated early to promote utilization of available ROM and to increase strength.

H. Grip strengthening can be initiated at 6 weeks postoperatively; however, if a concurrent tenolysis was performed, it is deferred until 8 to 10 weeks postoperatively.

II. Postoperative management of MCP capsulectomy

A. Begin AROM 1 to 3 days postoperatively as per doctor's orders. Active exercises should include blocked and full excursion flexion and extension.

B. PROM: instruction in *gentle* passive stretching.

C. Splinting

1. Instruction in skin care and routine checking for pressure areas in order to prevent skin breakdown.

2. Static splint MCPs placed near the limit of obtainable flexion with the wrist in extension to be used at night; this needs to be monitored closely and adjusted frequently as flexion increases; continue night splinting until ROM goals are met and maintained for a few weeks (Fig. 37-3).

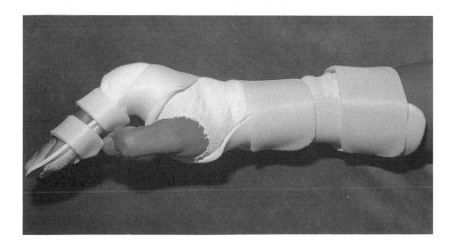

Fig. 37-3. Postoperative night positioning for MCP capsulectomy.

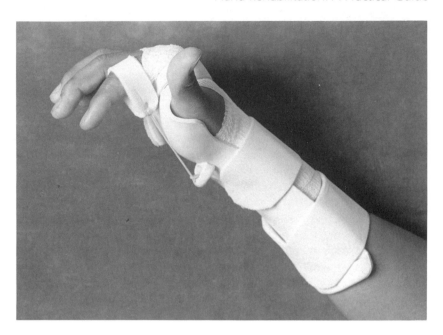

Fig. 37-4. Dynamic MCP flexion splint used intermittently during day.

3. Dynamic splinting to increase MCP flexion should be used intermittently during the day. Splint use should be followed by active exercise in order to help maintain gains in PROM achieved by splinting (Fig. 37-4).
4. If an extension lag is present, dynamic flexion splinting should be alternated with dynamic extension splinting (Fig. 37-5).
D. Functional activities should be promoted to utilize gains in ROM and to increase strength.
E. Muscle re-education of wrist extensors may be necessary as pa-

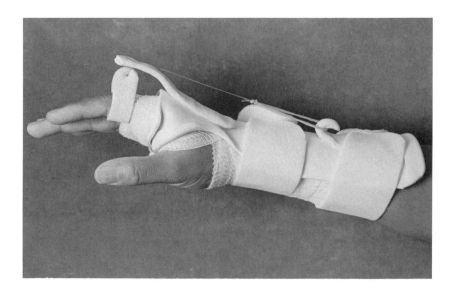

Fig. 37-5. Dynamic extension splint should be used during day if an extension lag is present.

tients may have been substituting their digital extensors for wrist extension and this pattern can contribute to stiffness in extension of MCPs and also interfere with grip strength.[2]

   F. Continuous passive motion (CPM) can be a useful adjunct to help decrease postoperative pain and edema while increasing PROM.

III. Postoperative management of PIP capsulectomy

   A. PIP capsulectomy secondary to extension contracture

     1. Dynamic flexion and extension splinting are alternated during the day (ratio of flexion versus extension splinting is determined by the available ROM).

     2. AROM should emphasize blocked active flexion and extension exercises.

     3. Static night splint position is determined by available range and anatomic structures involved.

   B. PIP capsulectomy secondary to flexion contracture

     1. Depending on the severity of the contracture and the surgeon's preferred method, the PIP joint may be pinned in extension postoperatively with initiation of exercise and splinting deferred until pin removal at 1 to 2 weeks postoperatively.

     2. The static splint maintains PIP joint extension at night and in between active exercise sessions (Fig. 37-6).

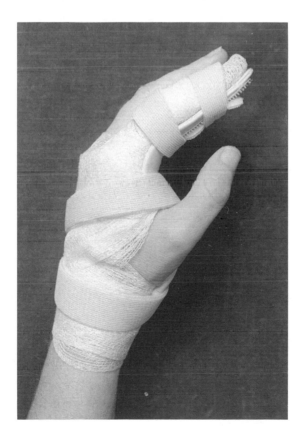

Fig. 37-6. Static PIP extension splint used at night and between active exercises.

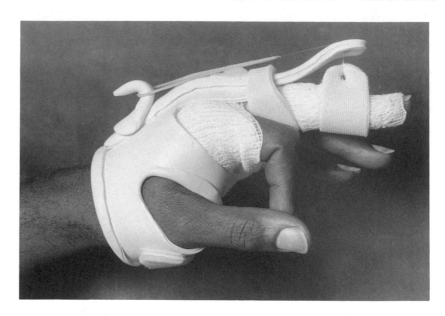

Fig. 37-7. Dynamic extension splint can be used during day for increasing extension.

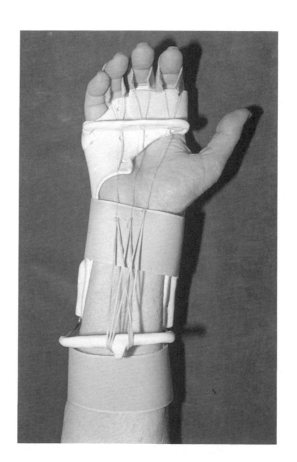

Fig. 37-8. Dynamic flexion splint can be used during day for increasing flexion.

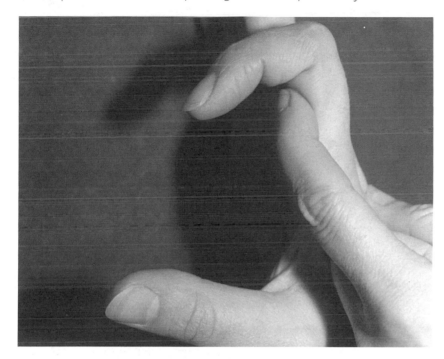

Fig. 37-9. Blocked ROM exercises should be included in exercise program.

3. Alternate dynamic extension and flexion splinting can be used during the day (as indicated by ROM) (Figs. 37-7 and 37-8).

4. An active exercise program should include blocked PIP flexion and extension (Fig. 37-9). If an extension lag is present it is important to protect it, via splinting, and prevent further loss of extension as ROM into flexion improves. Failure to monitor PIP joint extension closely can result in recurrence of the flexion contracture.

5. The oblique retinacular ligament may have become tight secondary to the flexion contracture and stretching exercises should be initiated (Fig. 37-10).

POSTOPERATIVE COMPLICATIONS

I. Infection
II. Limitations in ROM secondary to edema and/or pain
III. Weakness of previously adherent tendons
IV. Joint subluxation secondary to excessive ligament excision
V. Reflex sympathetic dystrophy (RSD)

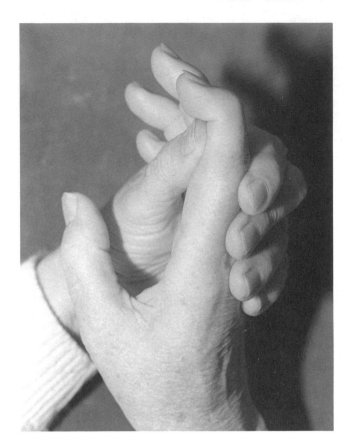

Fig. 37-10. Stretching exercise for oblique retinacular ligament.

EVALUATION TIMELINE

I. Preoperative evaluation 1 to 2 weeks before surgery to include
   A. AROM/PROM
   B. Grip and pinch strength
   C. Sensation
II. Postoperative evaluation
   A. Initial AROM postoperatively
   B. Weekly re-evaluation of AROM/PROM
   C. At 6 to 8 weeks: evaluation of ROM, sensation, and strength
      If a concurrent tenolysis was performed, evaluation of strength
      is deferred until 8 to 10 weeks postoperatively.

REFERENCES

1. Curtis RM: Capsulectomy of the interphalangeal joints of the fingers. J Bone
   Joint Surg (Am) 36:1219, 1954
2. Laseter G: Postoperative management of capsulectomies. p. 364. In Hunter

JM, Schneider LH, Mackin EJ, Callahan AD (eds): Rehabilitation of the Hand. 3rd Ed. CV Mosby, Baltimore, 1990
3. Gould JS, Nicholson BG: Capsulectomy of the metacarpophalangeal and proximal interphalangeal joints. J Hand Surg 4(5):482, 1979

SUGGESTED READINGS

McEntee P: Therapists management of the stiff hand. p. 328. In Hunter JM, Schneider LH, Mackin EJ, Callahan AD (eds). Rehabilitation of the Hand. 3rd Ed. CV Mosby, Baltimore, 1990
Young VL, Wray RC, Jr, Weeks PM: The surgical management of stiff joints in the hand. Plast Reconstr Surg 62:835, 1978
Flynn MD: Hand Surgery. 3rd Ed. William & Wilkins, Baltimore, 1982, p 335
Campbell's Operative Orthopaedics. 7th Ed. CV Mosby, St. Louis, 1987
Green DP (ed): Operative Hand Surgery. 2nd Ed. Churchill Livingstone, New York, 1988, p 537

Internal/External Fixation of Wrist and Distal Forearm Fractures

38

Linda Coll Ware

Joint congruency is essential to assure a good functional wrist. The fundamental goal of treating a wrist fracture is an accurate and stable reduction.[1] There are many techniques for fracture fixation outlined in the literature: percutaneous pin fixation, pins and plaster, closed reduction and external fixation, and open reduction and internal fixation.[1] Which technique a physician chooses depends upon many variables, including type of fracture, associated injuries, loss of bone substance, age and occupation of patient, and physician's surgical expertise.

Rehabilitation of wrist fractures begins immediately after fracture reduction and stabilization.[2] Internal fixation and dynamic external fixation enable early active motion of the wrist at week 1. External fixation does not allow wrist motion until as early as 6 weeks.

Open communication between physician and therapist is critical. Radiographic changes must be communicated to the therapist. Progressive therapy and strengthening should only be started after consulting the physician between 6 and 12 weeks.

Over a period of several months the patient progresses from active exercises to increasingly resistive activities. Steady improvement is expected for 8 to 12 months until full functional ability is achieved.[2]

DEFINITION

1. External fixation: a method of holding together the fragments of a fractured bone by employing transfixing metal pins through the fragments and a compression device attached to the pins outside the skin surface. The pins are removed at a later procedure when the fracture is healed.[3] (Figs. 38-1 and 38-2).

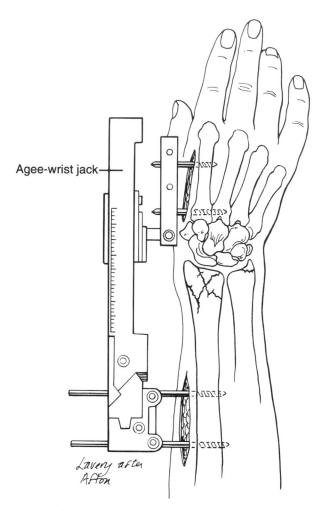

Agee-wrist jack——

Lavery after
Afton

Fig. 38-1. External fixation of fracture.

II. Internal fixation: any method of holding together the fragments of a fractured bone without the use of appliances external to the skin. After open reduction of the fracture, smooth or threaded pins, Kirschner wires (K-wire), screws, plates attached by screws, or medullary nails may be used to stabilize the fragments. In some instances the device is removed at a later operation, but sometimes it may remain in the body permanently[3] (Figs. 38-3 and 38-4).

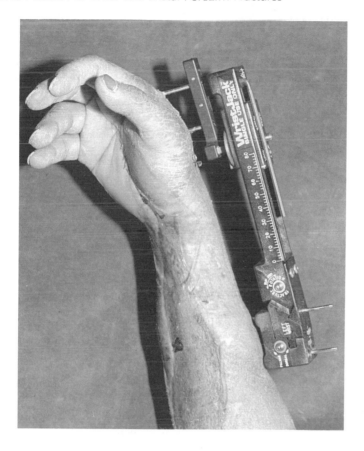

Fig. 38-2. External fixation of a distal forearm fracture.

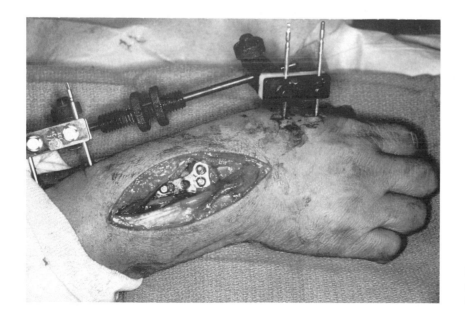

Fig. 38-3. Internal fixation may be used in combination with external device.

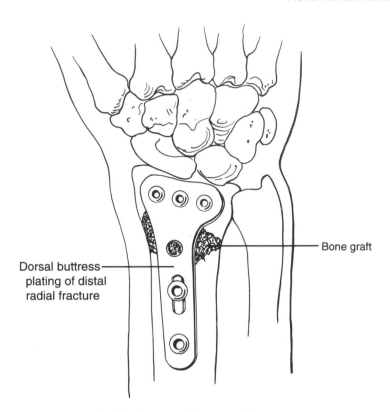

Fig. 38-4. Internal fixation of fracture.

TREATMENT AND SURGICAL PURPOSE

Many fractures of the distal radius and ulnar are unstable. Because the structure of the radius at this level is mostly cancelous, it will not easily stay reduced and may require some form of stabilization. The principal forms of stabilization are pins, bone plates, and external fixation devices. These may be used singly or in combination to achieve and maintain an acceptable reduction of the fracture. On occasion bone grafting to the radius may be necessary when these techniques are used in order that sufficient bone stock is present for strong healing. Combinations of fractures and dislocation of the carpal bones as well as the radius and ulnar occur and require accurate reduction and stabilization.

TREATMENT GOALS

I. Maintain full range of motion (ROM) of all uninvolved joints
II. Prevent wound or pin tract infection
III. Provide mobilization or immobilization of fixated joint as per fixation device
IV. Return to previous level of function

POSTOPERATIVE INDICATIONS/PRECAUTIONS FOR THERAPY

I. Indications
    Wrist fractures requiring internal or external fixation
II. Precautions
    A. Associated soft tissue loss
    B. Associated tendon injuries
    C. Associated nerve injuries

POSTOPERATIVE THERAPY

I. Therapy following internal fixation of wrist
    A. Week 1
        1. Thermoplastic splint to immobilize fixated fracture for amount of time directed by physician
            a. Thermoplastic splints are easy to remove for bathing or dressing changes if there is associated soft tissue loss
            b. If physician prefers a plaster cast, make sure uninvolved joints are not restricted
        2. Begin active ROM (AROM) of all uninvolved joints.
            Uninjured joint ROM can be enhanced by static and dynamic splinting.[2]
        3. Begin edema control.
    B. Week 2
        Begin gentle mobilization of wrist. Patient continues to wear splint when not exercising.
    C. Weeks 6 to 12
        When physician communicates radiographic union is clearly demonstrated, the splint may be discontinued and aggressive mobilization and strengthening can be started.
    D. Post 6 months
        Internal fixators may be removed 6 months after surgery or may remain in the body permanently.
II. Therapy following static external fixation of wrist
    A. Week 1
        1. Thermoplastic splint to immobilize fixated fracture for amount of time directed by physician. Splint may or may not be requested by physician.
            a. Splints are easy to remove for bathing or dressing changes if there is associated soft tissue loss.
            b. If physician prefers a plaster cast, make sure uninjured joints are not restricted.
        2. Begin AROM of all uninvolved joints.
            Uninjured joint ROM can be enhanced by static and dynamic splinting.[2]

   3. Begin edema control.
   4. Instruct patient on pin site care.
   B. Weeks 6 to 12
      Physician removes external fixator when radiographic union is demonstrated.
      1. A protective splint is applied to wrist.
      2. Mobilization progressing to strengthening can be started to regain full ROM and power.
III. Therapy following dynamic external fixation of the wrist[4]
   A. Week 1
      1. Begin active and active assisted wrist flexion from the neutral position.
      2. Begin AROM of all uninvolved joints.
      3. Begin edema control.
      4. Instruct patient on pin site care.
   B. Week 4
      Begin wrist extension and ulnar deviation.
   C. Weeks 8 to 10
      1. External fixation removed by physician.
      2. Progressive mobilization and strengthening of wrist started.

POSTOPERATIVE COMPLICATIONS

   I. Pin tract infection
  II. Pin site fracture
 III. Pin loosening
  IV. Osteoporosis
   V. Reflex sympathetic dystrophy (RSD)
  VI. Tendons adhering to internal fixation devices
 VII. Nerve impairment
VIII. Malunion
  IX. Refracture

EVALUATION TIMELINE

   I. Week 1
      A. AROM and passive ROM (PROM) measurements of all uninjured upper extremity joints
      B. Edema measurements
      C. Active and active assisted wrist flexion measurements if dynamic external fixation is used.
  II. Week 2
      AROM measurements of the internally fixated wrist
 III. Week 4
      ROM measurements of wrist extension and ulnar deviation if dynamic external fixation is used

IV. Weeks 6 to 12
   A. AROM measurements
   B. Grip strength measurements
   C. Pinch strength measurements
   D. Sensory screening

REFERENCES

1. Axelrod TS, McMurtry RY: Open reduction and internal fixation of comminuted, intra-articular fractures of the distal radius. J Hand Surg 15A:1, 1990
2. Melone Jr CP: Unstable fractures of the distal radius. p. 160. In Lichtmen DM (ed): The Wrist and Its Disorders. WB Saunders, Philadelphia, 1988
3. Glanze W (ed): Mosby's Medical, Nursing and Allied Health Dictionary. p. 454, 601. CV Mosby, St. Louis, 1989
4. Clyburn TA: Dynamic external fixation for comminuted intra-articular fractures of the distal end of the radius. J Bone Joint Surg 69(7):1110, 1987

SUGGESTED READINGS

Foster D, Kopta J: Update on external fixators in the treatment of wrist fractures. Clin Orthop 204:177, 1986
Freeland A, Jabaley M: Stabilization of fractures in the hand and wrist with traumatic soft tissue and bone loss. Hand Clin 4(3):425, 1988
Frykman G et al: Comparison of eleven external fixators for treatment of unstable wrist fractures. J Hand Surg 14A:247, 1989
Frykman GK, Nelson EF: Fractures and traumatic conditions of the wrist. p. 165. In Hunter JM, Schneider LH, Mackin EJ, Callahan AD (eds): Rehabilitation of the Hand. CV Mosby, St. Louis, 1984
Leung KS et al (ed): An effective treatment of comminuted fractures of the distal radius. J Hand Surg 15A:11, 1990
Riggs Jr SA, Cooney III WP: External fixation of complex hand and wrist fractures. J Trauma 23(4):332, 1983

Appendix 38-1

Wrist Fractures and Types of Fixation

Type of Fracture	Type of Fixation
A. Scaphoid fracture	Cast immobilzation Closed internal fixation Open internal fixation
B. Triquetrum fracture	Cast immobilization
C. Lunate fracture	Cast immobilization Closed internal fixation Open internal fixation
D. Hamate body fracture	Cast immobilization Closed internal fixation Open internal fixation
E. Trapezium fracture	Surgical reduction with internal fixation
F. Colles fracture (distal radius and ulna styloid)	Closed reduction with cast Closed reduction with internal fixation Open reduction internal fixation
G. Barton's fracture (distal radius)	Open reduction internal fixation with cast immobilization
H. Smith's fracture (distal radius)	Closed reduction with cast Closed reduction with internal fixation Open reduction internal fixation
I. Comminuted intra-articular fractures of distal radius	Dynamic external fixation External fixation Open reduction internal fixation
J. Combinations of distal forearm and carpal bone fractures	Combination of internal and external fixation. Closed and/or open reduction

Palmar Shelf Arthroplasty 39

Bonnie Aiello

The procedure palmar shelf arthroplasty is typically done to severely dislocated or subluxated, painful rheumatoid wrists. It is an attempt to reduce the joint, decrease pain, and maintain some motion at that joint while producing stability.

The carpus is reduced on a volar shelf formed by excision of a dorsal distal block of the radius.

Patients for whom this procedure is indicated have usually had the deformity for some time, causing tissue shortening. Radial shortening osteotomy, ulnar head resection, and carpal excision may all be utilized in order to reduce the joint. The joint capsule may be used as an interpositional graft.

Motion is then maintained at this fabricated joint. This is limited motion and should not be forced, as stability is very important and function does not require excessive motion.

Rehabilitation requires cast immobilization for 4 to 6 weeks followed by progressive motion and strengthening emphasizing function.

DEFINITION

Relocation of the carpus onto a volar fabricated shelf carved into the distal radius (Fig. 39-1)

SURGICAL PURPOSE

To gain joint stability and retain wrist motion with diminished pain. This operation is used almost exclusively in patients with rheumatoid arthritis where there is advanced loss of normal wrist architecture. A syno-

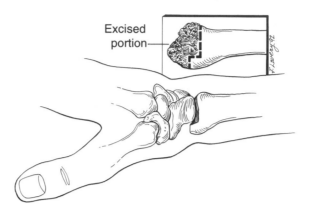

Fig. 39-1. Relocation of the carpus onto a volar fabricated shelf carved into the distal radius.

vectomy is performed, the volarly displaced carpus is perched on a small, surgically created shelf on the ventral cortex of the radius, and the entire configuration is pinned in place for 3 to 5 weeks to allow for adequate fibrous healing to occur.

TREATMENT GOALS

   I. Pain relief
  II. Wrist stability for function
 III. Increased motion
 IV. Reduction of the joint

POSTOPERATIVE INDICATIONS/PRECAUTIONS FOR THERAPY

  I. Indications
     A. Severe subluxation
     B. Dislocation
     C. Pain
     D. Rheumatoid arthritis
 II. Precautions
     A. Severe tissue shortening
     B. Articular surface distraction
     C. No concentrated effort made to get severe limits of flexion and extension since this jeopardizes stability.

POSTOPERATIVE THERAPY

Wrist splint in 20 degrees extension allowing full finger and thumb motion 4 to 6 weeks, then splint weaned progressively. Strengthening at 8 weeks.

POSTOPERATIVE COMPLICATIONS

I. Pain
II. Spontaneous fusion

EVALUATION TIMELINE

I. Postoperative
   A. Active range of motion (AROM): weeks 4 to 6
   B. Strength and passive range of motion (PROM): week 8

SUGGESTED READINGS

Albright J, Chase R: Palmar shelf arthroplasty of the wrist in rheumatoid arthritis. J Bone Joint Surg 52A(5):896, 1970

Gellman H, Rankin G, Brumfield R Jr: Palmar shelf arthroplasty in the rheumatoid wrist. J Bone Joint Surg 71A(2):23, 1989

Jackson I, Simpson RG: Interpositional arthroplasty of the wrist in rheumatoid arthritis. The Hand 2(2):169, 1979

Shoff N: Palmar shelf arthroplasty. J Bone Joint Surg 70A(9):1377, 1988

Proximal Row Carpectomy **40**

Bonnie Aiello

Injury to the proximal carpal row can lead to long-standing pain and disability. Wrist fusion is often offered to these patients but proximal row carpectomy is a valid option that can decrease pain and still maintain motion.

The triquetrum, lunate, and all or a piece of the scaphoid are removed. The distal carpus then articulates with the radius, not the ulna.

The surgery hinges on the fact that the distal pole of the capitate and the lunate fossa both be in good shape. This will be the major articulation of the wrist.

Postoperative therapy calls for approximately 1 month in a cast to provide stability and allow for healing. This is then followed by progressive motion and strengthening.

DEFINITION

Removal of the proximal row of carpal bones allowing the capitate to articulate with the lunate fossa (Fig. 40-1). Usually done in severe perilunate dissociation and Kienböck's disease to decrease pain and retain wrist motion.

SURGICAL PURPOSE

To relieve wrist pain, retain some wrist motion, and achieve joint stability. The proximal row includes the scaphoid, the lunate, and the triquetrum. The success of the procedure is dependent on good to excellent articular surfaces of the face of the capitate and the lunate fossa of the radius into which the capitate nestles.

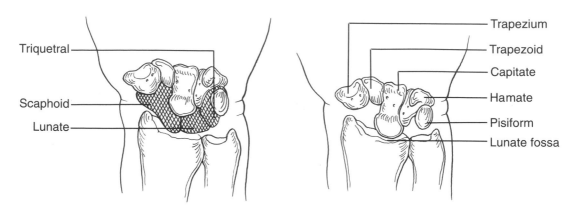

Fig. 40-1. Removal of the proximal row of carpal bones allowing the capitate to articulate with the lunate fossa.

TREATMENT GOALS

I. Decrease wrist pain
II. Maintain wrist motion 50 to 70 percent
III. Maintain strength 50 to 80 percent grip

POSTOPERATIVE INDICATIONS/PRECAUTIONS FOR THERAPY

I. Indications
    A. Long-standing perilunate dislocation
    B. Scaphoid malunion/nonunion
    C. Unsuccessful silastic implant
    D. Advanced Kienböck's disease
    E. Radiocarpal arthrosis
    F. Rheumatoid arthritis
    G. Spastic wrist contractures
II. Precautions
    Poor articular surface of proximal pole of capitate or lunate fossa

POSTOPERATIVE THERAPY

Bulky dressing with volar forearm plaster cast times 5 days. Cast times 4 weeks with range of motion (ROM) of fingers and thumb. May use cockup for support for 2 to 4 weeks. Cast removed week 4 and active ROM (AROM) started, progress to resistance.

POSTOPERATIVE COMPLICATIONS

  I. Pain
 II. Weakness
III. Limited ROM

EVALUATION TIMELINE

Postoperative
  I. Digital ROM day 1
 II. Wrist AROM week 4
III. Wrist passive ROM (PROM) week 6
IV. Strength week 6

SUGGESTED READINGS

Green D: Management of wrist problems. Hand Clin 163, 1987

Green D: Operative Hand Surgery p. 198. 2nd Ed. Vol. 1. Churchill Livingstone, New York, 1988

Green D: Operative Hand Surgery. p. 927. 2nd Ed. Vol. 2. Churchill Livingstone, New York, 1988

Inglis A, Jones E: Proximal row carpectomy for diseases of the proximal row. J Bone Joint Surg 59A(4):45, 1977

Jorgenson E et al: Proximal row carpectomy. J Bone Joint Surg 51A(6):1104, 1969

Nevaiser R: Proximal row carpectomy for posttraumatic disorders of the carpus. J Hand Surg 8(3):301, 1983

Tsuge K: Comprehensive Atlas of Hand Surgery. p. 207. Year Book Medical Publishers, New York, 1990

Wrist Arthrodesis 41

Beth Farrell

Total and intercarpal wrist arthrodesis surgery is a very successful reconstructive procedure for stabilizing the wrist.[1] Intercarpal arthrodesis is useful in treating carpal instability resulting from destruction of the carpus as seen in arthritis and advanced Kienböck's disease.[2] This is the surgery of choice when the patient's job requires some wrist mobility and the radiocarpal joint is "relatively free of arthritis involvement."[1]

Total wrist arthrodesis compromises motion for stability and, in most cases, pain relief. It is often performed as salvage surgery for other failed procedures and for heavy laborers with advanced radiocarpal instability.[1] The nondominant wrist is usually fused in the neutral position and the dominant hand is positioned in 10 degrees of extension and 5 degrees of ulnar deviation.[2]

The immobilization phase following surgery can lead to stiff uninvolved joints of the upper extremity. Therefore, one of the primary goals of therapy is to maintain full range of motion (ROM) of all uninvolved joints. This phase also contributes to upper extremity weakness and decreased endurance. Thus, once fusion is complete, it is important to begin general conditioning, strengthening, and instruction in compensatory techniques. These will enhance the patient's level of functioning for return to work and normal activities.

The therapist plays an important role in the success of wrist arthrodesis. Communication between the doctor and therapist in regard to the healing process is important in determining appropriate timing to initiate various phases of treatment. It should be emphasized that this protocol offers only guidelines, which may vary with each patient's particular condition.

DEFINITION

I. Total wrist arthrodesis: the surgical immobilization of the wrist joint. An iliac or distal radius bone graft is inserted with internal fixation to stabilize the wrist in the desired position (Fig. 41-1).

II. Intercarpal arthrodesis: the surgical partial immobilization of the wrist joint for treatment of carpal instability. An iliac or distal radius bone graft is used to replace the subchondral bone and articular cartilage is removed[3] (Fig. 41-2).

SURGICAL PURPOSE

To eliminate wrist pain, to correct joint instability with deformity and concurrent pain. It is done at the expense of wrist joint motion.

The limited wrist fusion applies to fusing two or more carpal bones together. The most common fusions involve the trapezium, scaphoid, and

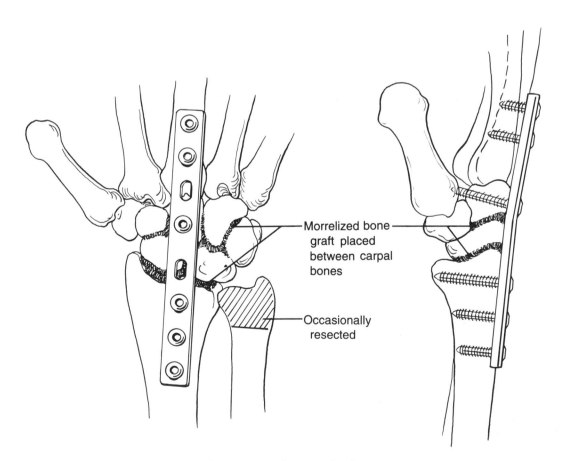

Morrelized bone graft placed between carpal bones

Occasionally resected

Fig. 41-1. Total wrist arthrodesis.

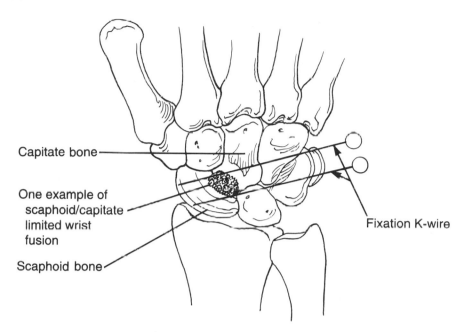

Fig. 41-2. Intercarpal arthrodesis.

trapezoid; the scaphoid and capitate; the lunate triquetrum, hamate, and capitate; and the triquetrum and lunate. Other combinations are possible. If a carpal bone is damaged, such as the scaphoid or lunate, these fusions may be performed to allow for replacement. The vacated abnormal bone is substituted with a Silastic implant or a tendon or fascial "anchovy," but stability is achieved.

The total wrist fusion is performed to stop wrist pain, increase strength along with endurance, and create joint stability. The techniques vary to accomplish this fusion that binds the radius to the carpus and metacarpals. Internal fixation is frequently used in the form of plates and screws or pins. The distal ulna may or may not be excised depending on the circumstances. Bone grafting from the iliac crest or another source is required. The average length of time for bony fusion is approximately 12 weeks. Another 12 weeks is usually necessary to reach maximum benefit.

TREATMENT GOALS

  I. Improve stability of the wrist
 II. Maximize ROM of wrist (if intercarpal arthrodesis)
III. Protect fusion
 IV. Control edema
  V. Minimize pain
 VI. Minimize adhesions
VII. Maintain ROM of uninvolved joints
VIII. Return patient to maximum level of functioning

INDICATIONS/PRECAUTIONS FOR SURGERY

I. Indications
   A. Intercarpal wrist arthrodesis[2]
      1. Localized arthritis of carpus
      2. Carpal instability
      3. Advanced Kienböck's disease
      4. As salvage surgery for partial carpal bone loss
      5. Sparing of midcarpal joints with destruction limited to radiocarpal area
   B. Total wrist arthrodesis
      1. Wrist pain and/or instability resulting from degenerative changes
      2. Heavy laborer with advanced radiocarpal joint destruction[1]
      3. As salvage surgery for failed procedures[1] (e.g., arthroplasties, partial wrist fusion)
      4. Paralysis of wrist with the potential for tendon reconstruction[1]
      5. Reconstruction following tumor resection
      6. Adolescent spastic hemiplegia with wrist flexion deformity[1]
      7. Wrist extensors are ruptured or nonfunctioning[2]
II. Precautions for therapy
   Partial arthrodesis: vigorous wrist exercise may exacerbate wrist pain[2]

POSTOPERATIVE THERAPY

The timetable below is only a guideline. It is important to consult with the patient's physician regarding surgical procedure performed, treatment goals, and healing status of the fused wrist.
I. Partial wrist arthrodesis
   A. Postoperative day 1 through entire rehabilitation program
      1. Maintain ROM of uninvolved joints
      2. Edema control
      3. Pain control as needed
   B. Cast immobilization for 8 to 10 weeks or until pins are removed (with delayed union or nonunion, immobilization time is increased).[4]
   C. Short arm splint or thumb spica splint (depending upon procedure) is applied for 2 to 3 weeks following cast removal[4] (Fig. 41-3).
      1. 8 to 10 weeks: initiate gentle active ROM (AROM) of wrist.[5] Avoid forced wrist motion.[2]
      2. Initiate scar management and edema control of wrist and digits.
   D. Once the fusion is complete and with the physician's consent, begin graded strengthening of the wrist and work hardening.[2]
II. Total wrist arthrodesis
   Postoperative therapy is essentially the same as intercarpal wrist arthrodesis; however, a total wrist arthrodesis is generally immobilized in a plaster cast for a longer period (e.g., 12 weeks).[1]

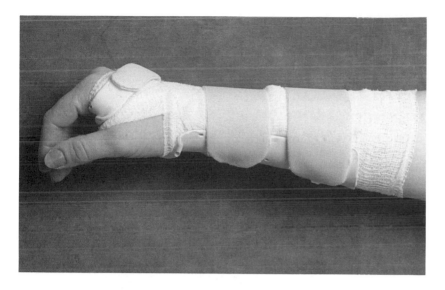

Fig. 41-3. Splint is applied after cast and/or pain removal.

POSTOPERATIVE COMPLICATIONS

   I. Pseudoarthrosis
  II. Fracture of healed fusion
 III. Nonunion
 IV. Deep wound infection
  V. Superficial skin necrosis
 VI. Vascular insufficiency/gangrene
 VII. Hematoma
VIII. Edema
 IX. Pain
  X. Transient median nerve or superficial radial nerve compression
 XI. Scar adhesions limiting tendon excursion

EVALUATION TIMELINE

  I. ROM
    A. Intercarpal wrist fusion
       1. 1 week postoperatively measure uninvolved upper extremity joints
       2. AROM of wrist once pins are removed
       3. Passive ROM (PROM): measured once fusion is complete
    B. Total wrist arthrodesis
       1 week postoperatively measure AROM and PROM of uninvolved upper extremity joints
  II. Sensory: Evaluate 1 week postoperatively. If deficits, evaluate at 1-month intervals following initial evaluation.
 III. Pain: Evaluate 1 week postoperatively and at every visit thereafter.

IV. Edema: Evaluate 1 week postoperatively and at every visit thereafter.
V. Scar formation: same as III and IV.
VI. Strength: Evaluate all upper extremity joints for strength once the fusion is complete.

REFERENCES

1. Dick HM: Wrist and intercarpal arthrodesis. p. 127. In Green DP (ed): Operative Hand Surgery. Vol. 1. Churchill Livingstone, New York, 1982
2. Nalebuff EA, Fatti JF, Weil CE: Arthrodesis of the rheumatoid wrist: indications and surgical technique. p. 365. In Lichtman DM: The Wrist and Its Disorders. WB Saunders, Philadelphia, 1988
3. Green DP: Carpal dislocations and instabilities. p. 925. In Green DP (ed): Operative Hand Surgery. 2nd Ed. Vol. 2. Churchill Livingstone, New York, 1988
4. Feldon P: Wrist fusions: intercarpal and radiocarpal. p. 446. In Lichtman DM (ed): The Wrist and Its Disorders. WB Saunders, Philadelphia, 1988
5. Watson HK, Black DM: Instabilities of the wrist. p. 103. In Taleisnick J (ed): Hand Clinics. Vol. 3. WB Saunders, Philadelphia, 1987

SUGGESTED READINGS

Clendenin MB, Green DP: Arthrodesis of the wrist—complications and their management. J Hand Surg 6:253, 1981
Fisk GR: The wrist: review article. J Bone Joint Surg 66B:401, 1984
Nalebuff EA, Fatti JF, Weil CE: Arthrodesis of the rheumatoid wrist: indications and surgical technique. p. 365. In Lichtman DM: The Wrist and Its Disorders. WB Saunders, Philadelphia, 1988

Reflex Sympathetic Dystrophy 42

Anne Edmonds

Reflex sympathetic dystrophy (RSD), which is described below, is a vasomotor dysfunction that can be localized to one area of an extremity or it can involve the entire extremity. Pain is the most outstanding complaint and swelling is the most outstanding physical feature.

RSD can be divided into three stages: acute, subacute, and chronic.

The acute stage begins at onset of injury and continues for approximately 3 months. Pain usually reaches its peak by the end of the first stage or beginning of the second stage. Swelling is apparent at this stage as is redness, increase in sweating, and limitation of motion secondary to the pain. X-rays may reveal demineralization and osteoporosis. The second stage usually extends from about the third to the ninth month with maximum pain and continued limited motion. The swelling is brawny and fixed. Redness begins to diminish during this stage and hyperhidrosis decreases as well. Stiffness continues with considerable periarticular thickening about the joints of the fingers. Atrophy of the skin and subcutaneous tissue along with palmar thickening of the longitudinal bands are noted in this stage. Osteoporosis is quite pronounced.

The third stage may last from many months to several years. The swelling and pain may subside but there continues to be considerable joint stiffness due to fibrotic changes. Skin color may appear pale and glossy. There is little hope of obtaining good motion at this stage.

DEFINITION

A vasomotor dysfunction that is characterized by very severe pain, swelling, stiffness, and discoloration (Fig. 42-1). It may appear following surgery, trauma, or local and systemic disease. It is variable in duration.

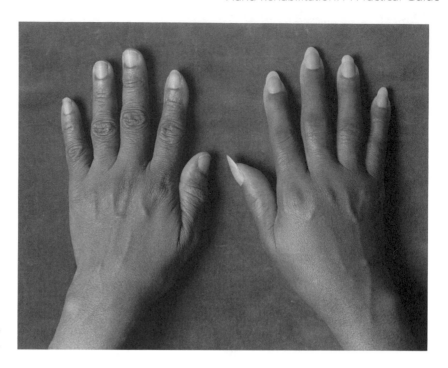

Fig. 42-1. RSD is a vasomotor dysfunction as seen in hand on right.

TREATMENT PURPOSE

The cause of RSD is poorly understood; however, the effects of this malady can be devastating to the patient and the involved part. It may occur following injury or surgery no matter how major or trivial. Its characteristics of pain, tenderness, swelling, and joint stiffness, when recognized or suspected, should be dealt with immediately to assure correction and restoration of maximum function. The early recognition of RSD leads to a better outcome of treatment. The diagnosis may sometimes be difficult and other pain-creating conditions must be ruled out so that the care of RSD patients can be maximized.

TREATMENT GOALS

To eliminate one of the three etiologic factors that must be present at the same time to produce RSD.

   I. Persistent painful lesion.
  II. Diathesis: two types
      A. Predisposition inherent characteristic, body trait
      B. Personality and psychological makeup (i.e., insecure, fearful, unstable)
 III. Abnormal sympathetic reflex to associated manifestations

NONOPERATIVE INDICATIONS FOR TREATMENT

I. Four cardinal signs and symptoms
    A. Pain
    B. Swelling
    C. Stiffness
    D. Discoloration
II. Secondary signs and symptoms that are most often but not always present
    A. Osseous demineralization
    B. Sudomotor changes
    C. Temperature changes
    D. Trophic changes
    E. Vasomotor instability
    F. Palmar fibromatosis

NONOPERATIVE THERAPY

I. Blocks
    A. Stellate: interrupted or continuous (Fig. 42-2)
    B. Bier
    C. Periodic perineural infusion

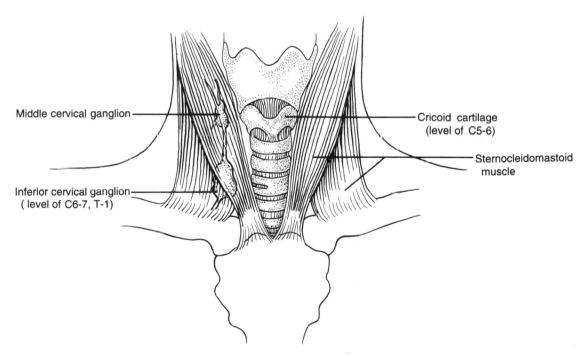

Fig. 42-2. Stellate ganglion block.

       D. Sympatholytic medication

       E. Sympathectomy

II. Therapy

   A. Acute stage

      1. Gentle active exercise and massage without pain; PROM with supervision

      2. Elevated hot packs

      3. Contrast baths

      4. High voltage galvanic stimulation (Fig. 42-3)

      5. Transcutaneous electrical nerve stimulation

      6. Splinting: protected, as indicated by patient's pain level

   B. Subacute, chronic

      1. All of the above mentioned in the acute stage

      2. Splinting: progressing to dynamic when tolerated by the patient

      3. Stress loading (Fig. 42-4).

      4. Functional activities

      5. Strengthening

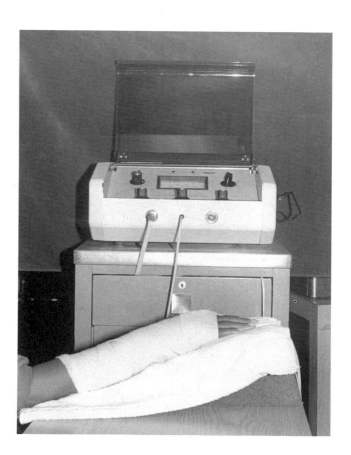

Fig. 42-3. High voltage galvanic stimulation treatment.

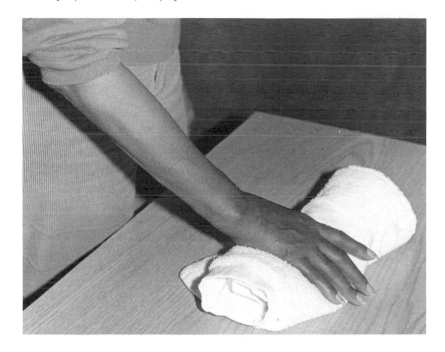

Fig. 42-4. Stress loading.

NONOPERATIVE COMPLICATIONS

I. High incidence of traumatic carpal tunnel syndrome
II. Late diagnosis and treatment can worsen and prolong the already established RSD

EVALUATION TIMELINE

I. Initial range of motion (ROM) measurements and once a month thereafter or before physician visit
II. Initial edema measurement and at each visit
III. Modalities indicated as tolerated by patient
IV. Splinting: protective/resting initially in functional position; work toward dynamic splinting as tolerated by patient

SUGGESTED READINGS

Lankford LL: Reflex sympathetic dystrophy. In Green DP (ed): Operative Hand Surgery. Vol. 1. Churchill Livingstone, New York, 1982
Lankford LL: Reflex sympathetic dystrophy. In Hunter JM, Schneider LH, Mackin EJ, Callahan AD (eds): Rehabilitation of the Hand. CV Mosby, St. Louis, 1990
Ramamurthy. Anesthesia. p. 23. In Green DP (ed): Operative Hand Surgery. Vol. 1. Churchill Livingstone, New York, 1982
Waylett-Rendall J: Therapists management of reflex sympathetic dystrophy. In Hunter JM, Schneider LH, Mackin EJ, Callahan AD (eds): Rehabilitation of the Hand. CV Mosby, St. Louis, 1990

Social Work Services

43

Ann Leman–Domenici

Since the beginning of the Raymond M. Curtis Hand Center, the clinical skills and services of social work have been an integral part of the interdisciplinary treatment offered to hand injured patients.

The social work function and role in this ambulatory, rehabilitative setting is a consultative one to staff, physicians, patients, and families. The primary focus is to explore the patients' and families' emotional reaction to the hand injury; what the injury means to them in terms of loss and change in their lives, and how they have typically coped with change. Also, specifically, asking the patient and family to clarify their understanding and expectations of treatment. According to Johnson:[1]

> The assessment also might involve exploration of how the injured person is handling grief. The person's sense of grief flows from the experience of loss, a loss of the use of one's hand if only temporary is significant. The loss triggers not only apprehensions over the future functioning of the hand but also the loss of employment, income and self-image as a productive, contributing person in a company or a family, if only for a short while. The stages of grief involving denial, depression and anger are important aspects to be assessed.[1]

Many psychosocial factors can be triggered as a result of a trauma or injury, including issues of body image, sexuality and self-identity, physical activity and pre-injury recreational/leisure time activities, changes in fulfilling social and familial roles, and responsibilities and employment issues.

The stated message in a psychosocial assessment is that the treatment team wants to learn what is the best way of treating the whole injured worker so that there will be a successful recovery and rehabilitation. The hand patient requires understanding, empathy, support, and education in establishing realistic goals.

The psychosocial support for the hand injured patient should begin as soon as possible following the injury. In order to accomplish this we utilize a screening questionnaire that is given to each patient by their hand therapist; the only exception is for one-time splint fabrications. The questionnaire was developed in collaboration with a community psychiatrist to assist the hand therapists early in treatment to identify patients who could benefit from social work referral and intervention.

The questionnaire includes the Holmes–Rahe stress producing life events check off list plus a 32-question inventory that asks about any pre-existing/concurrent medical problems, education and/or level of literacy, brief work history and job satisfaction ratios, relationship and/or marriage history, family/friend support system, transient or stability of residence, previous mental health treatment, symptoms of depression, alcohol/drug usage including prescribed medication, difficulty with the law, and any job-related problems due to substance abuse.

DEFINITION

Referrals for social work services are typically received from physicians, hand therapists, work adjustment therapists, and rehabilitation nurses, through direct referrals, and/or the weekly social work meeting.

I. Important indicators for referral
   A. Adjustment to injury issues
   B. Alcohol/drug abuse and/or recovery issues
   C. Anxiety
   D. Depression
   E. Specific diagnoses
      1. Reflex sympathetic dystrophy (RSD) syndrome
      2. Traumatic upper extremity amputation
      3. Chronic pain
      4. Conversion reactions
      5. Factitious disorder
   F. Family problems
   G. Financial issues
   H. High stressors
   I. Lack of social supports
   J. Marital problems
   K. Previous psychiatric treatment
   L. Post-traumatic stress disorders
   M. Transportation to treatment issues

ASSESSMENT

The social worker will complete a comprehensive written psychosocial assessment, including the following information:
   I. The presenting problem as perceived by the patient
   II. Insurance coverage (Worker's Compensation claim, Medicare, medical assistance, self-pay, commercial insurance), financial and legal status

III. Understanding of diagnosis, cause of symptoms, and expectations
IV. Patient's support network, family composition, family/marital status
V. Education level, work history, current job, and length of employment
VI. Current affective and cognitive functioning
VII. Stressors and emotional state
VIII. Current medications
IX. Alcohol/drug usage
X. Activities of daily living (ADL): What is a typical day like?
XI. Prior mental health treatment

In addition to the screening questionnaire and the clinical interview, at times, the Minnesota Multiphasic Personality Inventory (MMPI) is utilized to assist in formulating a treatment plan and obtaining authorization from the insurance carriers for treatment recommendations. The MMPI is explained to the hand patient as an objective standard measure that will potentially verify symptoms that were discussed in the clinical interview, in order to support the recommendation for a psychiatric evaluation.

The social worker has the patient complete the MMPI and forwards the raw data to a psychiatrist who scores and interprets the information.

Once the assessment is complete, the social worker will collaborate with the patient, the hand therapist, the physician, and the rehabilitation specialist in order to initiate a treatment plan for the patient, to include appropriate plan of action steps and appropriate referrals. This is not a passive process in which the patient is the receiver of the social worker's treatment, but an active process of cooperation.

Additionally, the hand-injured patient's spouse or significant other is invited to participate in the sessions. At times a telephone interview is the next best alternative, to obtain information and enlist support toward the recommended plan of treatment. Especially if the recommendation is for a psychiatric evaluation, at times the spouse or significant other needs assistance as well.

TREATMENT GOALS

Treatment goals will vary depending on the identified and agreed upon problem. Diagnostic indicators for specific problems will be presented utilizing the indicators for referral list.

I. Adjustment to injury issues
   A. The treatment goal is to provide information, referral, and emotional support, and to advocate on behalf of the patient. Below are a few examples.
      1. Basic information on the Workers Compensation system is provided.
      2. Overall orientation to the Hand Center's purpose and philosophy, with clarification of the patient and institution's roles and responsibilities.

      3. Information and referral to community resources as appropriate.
         a. Adult literacy and/or GED program to improve skills and to provide a productive, structured activity.
         b. Encourage volunteer employment to reduce boredom, increase activity level, and promote self-esteem.
         c. Referral to the State Division of Vocational Rehabilitation.
         d. Recommend participation in a senior center for social support and to reduce isolation and symptoms of depression for senior citizens.
         e. Referral to support groups.

II. Alcohol/drug abuse/addictions (eating, smoking, gambling)
    The treatment goal is to identify the problem, educate the patient about the treatment available, and make a recommendation for treatment to the patient and physician. Also to reinforce and support the program of recovery being used.
    A. Documented use (e.g., emergency room) of alcohol/drugs when the injury occurred.
    B. Alcohol being utilized to self-medicate for pain management.
    C. Use of prescription narcotics for more than a 2- to 3-month period of time postinjury and/or surgery.
    D. Patient arrives for hand treatment under the influence.
    E. Self-identified recovering alcoholic or addict who is working a 12-step program. The stress of the injury and rehabilitation can make the individual high risk for a relapse.
    F. Cigarette addiction that is compromising the physical outcome of the hand.
    G. Gambling behavior that is interfering with financial resources to engage or follow through with treatment.

III. Anxiety
    The treatment goal is to identify the symptoms and provide education and treatment recommendations. Anxiety disorders are treated by a combination of cognitive behavior therapy and medication and usually require a psychiatric evaluation.
    A. Phobic disorder: The essential feature is the fear of an activity, situation, or object that results in a desire to avoid the same. When the avoidance behavior or fear is a significant source of distress and interferes with social or role functioning, treatment is indicated.
    B. Panic disorder: The essential feature is sudden onset of intense apprehension, fear, or terror, associated with feelings of impending doom. Symptoms include dyspnea, palpitations, chest pain, dizziness or unsteady feelings, sweating, faintness, trembling or shaking, hot/cold flashes.

IV. Depression
    The treatment goal is to identify the symptoms, educate the patient about available treatment, and make a recommendation for

treatment to the patient and physician. Typical treatment involves medication and psychotherapy. Symptoms to be aware of include:

    A. Loss of interest or pleasure in all or almost all usual activities, withdrawal from family and friends

    B. Appetite disturbance, either extreme: increased appetite and weight gain or loss of appetite and weight loss

    C. Sleep disturbance

    D. Concentration difficulties, increased forgetfulness

    E. Suicidal ideation

V. Specific diagnoses

    A. RSD syndrome/chronic pain: The treatment goal is to identify symptoms of depression and educate the patient about the benefits of antidepressants in pain management and the symptoms of depression. Also to refer to local RSD support group.

    B. Traumatic upper extremity amputation. The treatment goal is to identify symptoms of loss, anger, and depression and to provide adjustment to injury counseling. Referrals to the Amputee Association of America is a standard procedure. Psychiatric evaluation is often indicated.

    C. Posttraumatic stress disorder (PTSD): recognition that the hand patient experienced an event outside the range of usual human experience. The treatment goal is to return the hand-injured worker to full psychological functioning or as close as possible through psychotherapy and a desensitization program.

       The five major characteristics of PTSD include

      1. The traumatic event is persistently re-experienced.

      2. Recurrent and intrusive distressing recollection of the event.

      3. Recurrent distressing dreams of the event.

      4. Sudden acting or feeling as if the traumatic event were recurring (flashback episodes).

      5. Persistent avoidance of stimuli associated with the traumatic event.

VI. Conversion reactions

    The treatment goal is to identify symptom and related issues and refer for psychiatric evaluation. The main symptoms is a loss or change in physical functioning that suggests a physical disorder but which is an expression of a psychological conflict or need. The disturbance is not under the voluntary control of the patient.

VII. Factitious disorder with physical symptoms

    The treatment goal is to identify symptoms and refer for psychiatric evaluation. The essential feature is the presentation of physical symptoms that are not real. An example would be self-inflicted tourniqueting of the upper extremity.

VIII. Family problems

    The treatment goal is to identify and educate the patient about available resources.

    A. History of physical, sexual, emotional abuse

    B. Bereavement issues when there is a loss of a family member

IX. Financial issues

The treatment goal is to identify the problem and the potential resources and make the necessary referrals.

A. Referral to the Department of Social Services for medical assistance, general public assistance, food stamps
B. Referral to the internal mechanisms of the hospital for financial assistance

X. Stressors are high

The treatment goal is to identify the stressors and educate the patient in stress management techniques using a cognitive behavioral approach.

XI. Lack of social supports

The treatment goal is to engage the patient in recognizing the problem and to brainstorm solutions.

A. Encourage and direct the patient to volunteer in some capacity.
B. Encourage the patient to participate in church-related activities.
C. Encourage participation in a support group.

XII. Marital problems

The treatment goal is to identify couples issues as the problem and to refer couples for counseling.

XIII. Previous and/or current psychiatric treatment

The treatment goal is to obtain the name of the previous or current treating mental health professional and their phone number from the patient. If behavioral changes are observed during the course of hand treatment, contact can be initiated with this resource person.

XIV. Transportation to treatment

The treatment goal is to facilitate the patient's hand treatment. This could mean contacting the insurance carrier and explaining the problem and negotiating a solution.

REFERENCE

1. Johnson RK: Psychological evaluation of patients with industrial hand injuries. Occup Injuries 3:567, 1986

SUGGESTED READINGS

Bear-Lehman J: Factors affecting return to work after hand injury. Am J Occup Ther 37(3):189, 1983

Cone J, Hueston JT: Psychological aspects of hand injury. Med J Austral 1:104, 1974

Grant GH: The hand and the psyche. J Hand Surg 5:417, 1980

Grunert BK, Devine CA, Matloub HS et al: Sexual dysfunction following traumatic hand injury. Ann Plast Surg 1:46, 1988

Grunert BK, Devine CA, McCallum-Burke S et al: On-site work evaluation: desensitizing for avoidance reactions following hand trauma. J Hand Surg 14B:239, 1989

Grunert BK, Matloub HS, Sanger JR, Yousif NJ: Treatment of post traumatic stress disorder after work related hand trauma. J Hand Surg 15A3:511, 1990

Grunert BK, Smith CJ, Devine CA et al: Early psychological aspects of traumatic hand injury. J Hand Surg (Br) 13B:177, 1988

Hansen F. Psychiatric aspects of the hand patient: their importance in patient assessment. American Physical Therapy Assoc. Hand Section Newsletter, Volume I:4, November 1983

Lee PWH, Ho ESY, Tsang AKT, Chang JCY: Psychosocial adjustment of victims of occupational hand injuries. Soc Sci Med 20(5):493, 1985

Louis DS, Lamp M, Greene T: The upper extremity and psychiatric illness. J Hand Surg 10A(5):687, 1985

Mendelson R, Burech J, Polack EP, Kappel D: The psychological impact of traumatic amputations, a team approach: physicians, therapists and psychologist. Occup Injuries 3:577, 1986

Montague J, Rosner, Stein V: Social work's role in managing chronic pain. Dimens Health Serv 66(3):23, 1989

Tomlinson WK: Psychiatric complications following severe trauma. J Occup Med 7:454, 1974

Index

Page numbers followed by an f indicate figures, and those followed by a t indicate tables.